AF361261

A CHORUS OF UNHEARD VOICES

A Chorus of Unheard Voices

The Invisible Work of Medical Education

EDITED BY ANNA MACLEOD
AND LARA VARPIO

UNIVERSITY OF TORONTO PRESS
Toronto Buffalo London

© University of Toronto Press 2026
Toronto Buffalo London
utppublishing.com
Printed in Canada

ISBN 978-1-4875-7226-6 (cloth) ISBN 978-1-4875-7315-7 (EPUB)
ISBN 978-1-4875-7269-3 (PDF)

Library and Archives Canada Cataloguing in Publication

Title: A chorus of unheard voices : the invisible work of medical education /
   edited by Anna MacLeod and Lara Varpio.
Names: MacLeod, Anna, 1976– editor | Varpio, Lara, editor
Description: Includes bibliographical references.
Identifiers: Canadiana (print) 20260123897 | Canadiana (ebook) 20260123900 |
   ISBN 9781487572266 (cloth) | ISBN 9781487572693 (PDF) |
   ISBN 9781487573157 (EPUB)
Subjects: LCSH: Medical education. | LCSH: Medical personnel. |
   LCSH: Medical colleges – Administration. | LCSH: Teaching hospitals –
   Administration.
Classification: LCC R735 .C46 2026 | DDC 610.71/1 – dc23

Cover design: Sebastian Stachowski
Cover image: Shutterstock.com/design36

The manufacturer's authorised representative in the EU for product safety
is Mare Nostrum Group B.V., Doelen 72, 4831 GR Breda, The Netherlands.
Email: gpsr@mare-nostrum.co.uk

We wish to acknowledge the land on which the University of Toronto Press
operates. This land is the traditional territory of the Wendat, the Anishnaabeg,
the Haudenosaunee, the Métis, and the Mississaugas of the Credit First Nation.

University of Toronto Press acknowledges the financial support of the
Government of Canada, the Canada Council for the Arts, and the Ontario Arts
Council, an agency of the Government of Ontario, for its publishing activities.

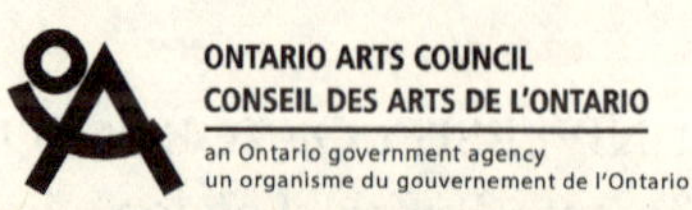

This book, and everything really, is dedicated to Mary Claire, Andrew, and Marcus. Wherever life takes you, may your ideas always be valued and your voices always heard.

Contents

Part Two: Evidence Assembly

Part Three: Institutional Concerns

Conclusion

Illustrations

Preface

Everything we knew for sure about our work had been turned upside down. In the early days of the COVID-19 pandemic when, depending on which part of the world you were in, lockdowns or shelter-in-place restrictions were still very much in place, work was changing too. We worked at home, but we were uncertain and, while we may not have used the language at the time, lonely – grieving the way things were and missing what work used to be. Amid a sea of very real pandemic-related concerns was one more: that we may never go back to the way things were at work.

But we adapted. We figured out how to do it all, but differently, in this new, digitized, and distant context. We made it happen, despite a quiet but persistent sadness because – who would have guessed it – *we missed going to work*. The social side of it. Our work friends. The physical spaces of our offices. The change of scenery. The people we'd smile at in the corridor. Conversations in the coffee line with people we'd never plan a meeting with. Of course, we stayed in touch with close colleagues through online connections and through awkward attempts at informal digital gatherings. But despite our efforts, it wasn't the same. In particular, the tools of video conferencing, which were designed to facilitate a certain type of connection, mediated all our interactions. Made it all feel more formal and structured. Encouraged us to stick to the agenda and end on time. We missed the stories. The laughs and encouragement.

As the initial "two weeks to stop the spread" evolved into months (and eventually years), the idea for this book came to us. If we can't see people incidentally, let's do it on purpose. Let's create a space in which our friends and colleagues can tell their stories, share their expertise. Let's not only see them. Let's really listen, too. And so, we conceptualized this book as a chorus of unheard voices. A place in which we can acknowledge and celebrate the complexity of medical education: the people working together to educate physicians – the people whose voices we rarely hear.

And so, we begin first and foremost by thanking and celebrating the incomparable Anne Mahalik. It's hard to write a "thank you" like this without sounding clichéd – but Anne really was the centre of our little universe as this book came together. While Anna and Lara were *idea* people, Anne was the *get organized and make it happen* person. Much more than our editorial associate, Anne was a provider of memes, a sounding board, a voice of reason, and a friend whose ideas always made things better. Her expertise and attention to detail are woven throughout this book. Truly, without Anne, this book simply would never have come into existence.

We also want to thank the authors who contributed to each chapter – the clinicians who explained why these roles are important to medical education, the scholars who placed this work in the context of current literature, and the individuals who shared their narratives illustrating what it is actually like to do this vital work. It would not have been possible to create such a powerful text had it not been for your energies, support, and candour. Also, we think our friend Adina Kalet for believing in our idea and helping us see the possibilities.

We lost our colleague and friend Rob Sandeski while this book was in development. Rob co-authored the chapter on anatomy technicians. He was a brilliant educator and innovator, and an all-around wonderful guy. We're sorry Rob didn't have the chance to see the book in print, but we know he would be proud.

On a personal note, Anna thanks the MacLeods, Heightons, and Muzikas – especially Jo-Anne and Gregor (aka Bucky and Nan), Pete and Aseil, and Marg and Jerry – for their constant encouragement and interest in her work, even when she says things like "sociomaterially mediated practices." She is grateful for the friendship of Paula Cameron and Olga Kits and has every intention of someday getting matching "Crushin' It" sweatbands. The biggest thank you of all goes to Greg and his incredibly generous soul for being the perfect partner to walk through life with – and for always finding the gluten-free bakeries along the way. And to Mary Claire for knowing exactly who she is, and for being a source of endless joy as she cartwheels bravely through life.

Lara thanks Suzanne Thorpe, Ebru Kuran, and Anne Mandeville who, across miles of walking and talking during the pandemic, became the sisters she'd dreamed of having. They are the unheard voices who enable so much of Lara's life – who always know where the best take-out dinners can be found, who have the email of an interior designer who helps the colour blind, and who will teach you how to cook a simple meal so that dinner is no longer referred to as "the five o'clock miracle." She also thanks the three essential men in her life: Johan, who is the ballast (and on-board entertainment) to the ship of life, and Andrew and Marcus, who consistently prove that, if you're lucky, your children embody the best of you and then outperform and outclass you in every single way.

Finally, we thank Canadian pop legend Corey Hart. Just trust us on this. And don't masquerade with the guy in shades, oh no.

Introduction

1 The Song Begins: A Chorus of Unheard Voices

ANNA MACLEOD AND LARA VARPIO

Medical schools are fascinating places. Over the years, they've captured our collective imagination. On television (*Scrubs, The Royal Flying Doctor Service*), in the movies (*Patch Adams, Red Beard*), and in print (*The House of God, Bloodletting and Miraculous Cures*), depictions of medical schools abound. They are hallowed places to which only a privileged few – the brightest and best – gain access. Medical educators are popularly imagined as serious senior professors, genius research scientists, or quirky-but-gifted clinicians, all of whom are entrusted with a single but significant job: preparing the next generation of physicians for practice.

Why this fascination with medical education? Of course, the broad medical field is inherently dramatic, with life-and-death scenarios taking place every day, providing rich fodder for storytelling – whether it's a complex surgical procedure or a challenging diagnosis. The characters populating these fictional medical schools are compelling. These are highly intelligent people who have already mastered or will eventually master the mysteries of our bodies. Guided through their education by savvy clinician teachers, they will come to know and understand the complex things happening both on and under our skin. And let us never forget the most important people in these dramas – the patients who ask for help. Their stories are part of the complex narratives that entwine all these people together.

These stories are also set in highly charged contexts. Hospitals and medical schools are large organizations brimming with political agendas, financial aspirations, and civic duties. High-stakes exams need to be passed. Babies will be birthed. Love may be kindled. Death is ever present. Clearly, medicine and medical dramas offer glimpses into the inner workings of the human body, interpersonal relationships, and social agendas. Portrayed on the screen and in text, physicians – and physicians in training – are often portrayed as heroes, strong characters who, while flawed, seem to be able to come through to solve mysteries, make diagnoses, and save lives.

While some of the popular media imagery from the fictional world of medical education holds true – the genius clinicians, high-pressure atmospheres, and the politics of hospitals are, in fact, part of medical education in the real world. But these portrayals offer only a highly edited (and even airbrushed) view of the everyday work of a real-life medical school. Perhaps most notably, they tend to ignore the many people involved in medical education whose skill sets, expertise, and behind-the-scenes work is essential to keeping medical schools and academic teaching hospitals running. So, before the serious senior professor was ever able to deliver an inspiring lecture, she was likely a research assistant supporting the research of another professor. Before that lecture could be given, an educational specialist planned the curriculum that called for the lecture. Someone else mapped the content of that lecture to learning objectives to ensure the school was meeting accreditation requirements. Someone else scheduled the lecture within a logistically complex curriculum. Someone else booked the lecture hall. Someone made sure that the room was clean, safe, and warm. Someone else pivoted the lecture from an in-person setting to an online space when COVID-19 hit. Someone else helped the professor embed a video into their PowerPoint. And the story goes on.

While television, movies, and books offer medical education imagery that focuses on the high-profile work of professors, researchers, and clinicians, those of us who make our living in medical schools know that our communities are composed of a multitude of people with different roles, some of which may not be surprising (financial and administrative roles, for example), but some of which are quite surprising (such as acting and embalming skills). For a variety of reasons, the skills and talents of these workers have remained largely unrecognized and underappreciated. We believe these invisible workers, and their commitment to excellence in their respective roles, are a large part of what make medical schools places of character, caring, and ultimately, competence. And for that reason, this book is a deliberate effort to offer a microphone so that we can hear their voices.

What Is the (Sociology of) Work of Medical Education?

What do we mean by work? Formally, work can be described as any activity that involves the expenditure of effort, physical or mental, in order to produce something: goods, services, or in our case, a physician.[1] It is typically performed in exchange for payment or some other form of compensation and is shaped by social and cultural factors including things like gender, race, social class, and globalization. Work, whatever the context, is an important part of social life and has significant impacts on individuals, families, and communities.

The work of medical education ultimately focuses on educating physicians – both future and current physicians – but certainly, such a broad statement obscures the huge diversity of tasks associated with this important work. And, of course, the concept of work is a central organizing feature for anyone working in the field of medical education: we engage in workplace-based education.[2] That is, medical education takes place not only in classrooms but also in hospitals, clinics, and community settings – real workplaces where patients are treated and lives are at stake. These learning environments are richly textured and inherently social. Workplace-based learning (WBL) refers to educational experiences that unfold in authentic clinical settings where learners engage in patient care under supervision, develop professional identity, and participate in the real-world practice of medicine.[3] This kind of learning is deeply relational and situational – shaped not only by clinical knowledge and skill, but also by the social norms, organizational cultures, and power dynamics of healthcare institutions.[4] Importantly, WBL relies on an extensive scaffold of invisible work: from clinical preceptors offering informal coaching while managing patient loads, to unit clerks orienting learners to workflow, to patients generously sharing their time and stories. We educate future physicians for what will become their life's work. We send them off to workplaces to learn and practise. We assess them on their ability to function professionally. But we rarely consider the infrastructures of human effort that make these assessments possible.

The sociology of work is a thriving academic discipline that addresses the complexities of work and work-related activities.[5-7] Sociologists who study work have helped us think more deeply about how work is organized, how it shapes society, and how it affects all of us. Their contributions have given us a language to make sense of a number of important concepts to consider in the broad realm of medical education. These include a wide range of topics, including things like the impact of unions and workers' rights, and a focus on working conditions and fair compensation. While these seem like considerations that are distinct from the enterprise of medical education, we are currently feeling the impact of these contributions as we continue to wrestle with resident working-hours limitations[8] and bear witness to ongoing junior doctors' strikes in the United Kingdom.[9] Sociologists studying work have also encouraged us to attend to issues of globalization. They've explored how the international nature of higher education has created new types of workers, for example, international medical graduates,[10] who are now commonly contributing to our medical education work. They've also studied new forms of work in which some academics find themselves, such as telecommuting and the gig economy.[11] Even Marxist critiques of capitalism, based in the sociology of work, have entered our collective consciousness as we examine the medical machine and how pressures to manage volume and meet quotas, in both clinical and academic work, lead to alienation and burnout.[12]

Clearly, we have much to learn from the sociology of work, and insights from this discipline have influenced current medical education conversations. However, in this volume we have chosen to centre concepts that have yet to be fulsomely embraced in our field: the division of labour[13] and social stratification.[14] What do these ideas mean, and why do they matter in medical education? In its simplest form, the division of labour refers to how work becomes divided and specialized in society, with certain tasks being recognized as prestigious and important and others less so. Building on this concept, social stratification addresses the ways in which society is organized into hierarchical layers based on social class, race, gender, and other factors. Different occupations and industries are associated with different levels of status and prestige.

Along with the division of labour and social stratification comes the concept of invisible work, which is the cornerstone concept of this volume – the idea that some of the essential work happening in medical schools and academic teaching hospitals, while indispensable, is pervasively underappreciated and remains largely off our radars. Rarely, if ever, do administrative assistants managing conflicts, librarians coordinating searches, or planners organizing a conference figure into the fast-paced medical dramas we see represented in popular media, despite the essentialness of their work. Our volume, then, is a deliberate step away from invisibility. A podium, with a spotlight. An invitation to hear stories and learn about skill sets we may have previously taken for granted.

Invisible Workers and Invisible Work

Let's unpack the concept of invisible work, since it is critical to the chapters that will follow. Simply put, this is the kind of work that is so much a part of the background that we rarely think about it or stop to pay attention. Maybe invisible isn't exactly the right word because these are things that are see-able. But we have to make a concerted effort to see them – they can easily evade our eye if we're not deliberate in our efforts to notice them.

Susan Leigh Star and Anslem Strauss[15] used the term invisible work to refer to the often-unnoticed effort required to maintain social structures in any given organization. They acknowledged that much of the work that keeps organizations running smoothly, including things like emotional labour (e.g., a research assistant may need to control their emotions and react calmly despite dealing with a principal investigator who has been rude or dismissive of their work), support work (e.g., an administrative assistant comforts an upset learner who is angry about their exam results) and administrative tasks (e.g., an administrator surfs the Internet endlessly to find the best sale price for materials in an effort to shrink costs in an era of decreasing budgets). These are all essential aspects of what makes medical education happen, for better or for worse; however, these efforts are largely invisible. They take place "backstage,"[16] and because of this, these tasks become taken for granted, their value poorly (if ever) recognized.

It's difficult to account for the abundance of invisible tasks that take place in a medical school without noting their gendered, raced, and classed nature. Over the years, the sociology of work has helped us to uncover how work is organized and controlled by larger social structures, such as gender and class relations, and how these, in turn, shape the experiences of workers. It has been a powerful tool for exploring how things like gender relations and norms influence the types of jobs that men and women are typically assigned, and how certain jobs are not only gendered, but also classed, raced, … and the list goes on.

In medical schools, and many other realms, much of the invisible work falls to people from traditionally marginalized or undervalued groups, including women, people of colour, immigrants, the working poor, and others. For example, in our field, women and people of colour are more likely to perform those undervalued tasks we described above.[17] These individuals engage in forms of emotional labour, providing support to others, and doing underappreciated – but essential – administrative tasks, while men and white people continue to be more likely to hold positions of authority and decision-making power.[18]

This disparity continues. The legacy of discrimination and exclusion in healthcare influences work in medical schools and academic teaching hospitals. People from equity-deserving groups have well-documented challenges accessing healthcare and employment opportunities.[19] They continue to be stereotyped and pigeonholed into certain roles.[20] Despite decades of social movements, women are still assumed to be better at providing emotional support and nurturing care,[21] while people of colour are still often assumed to be more "hands-on" and physically capable.[22] These stereotypes, in turn, can lead to a disproportionate representation in certain, lower-visibility roles, such as standardized patients or clinical skills instructors.[23]

While we applaud medical schools around the world in their efforts to address equity issues, there is a tremendous amount of work still to do, which is represented in workplace systems and structures that must adapt. This issue has manifested in a variety of ways, including as a lack of resources to support the recruitment and retention of people from underrepresented groups into leadership roles,[24] as well as a lack of recognition of the "minority tax,"[25] which refers to the extra responsibilities and burdens placed on individuals from marginalized groups in educational or workplace settings (such as extra time spent serving on diversity committees or mentoring other students or employees who are also from equity-deserving groups). All of this perpetuates a hierarchy of labour in which the expertise, skill, and contributions of people from equity-deserving groups remain undervalued and undercompensated[26] – in other words, invisible.

Being an invisible worker has been shown again and again to be exhausting.[15] It has been linked to burnout and stress, particularly for those who are doing the work without recognition or appropriate compensation.[27] This, in turn, can have serious implications for the individuals, but also for the broader institutions of medical education as they struggle with turnover and a sense of low morale.[28] And so the cycle continues.

How do we address it? In their seminal work, Star and Strauss argued that making the invisible visible is essential as we work towards healthier, happier, and more sustainable workplaces. And so, our book is a testament to the many unrecognized people of medical education. To their invisible expertise and their long hours spent in service to medical education's missions. To the open doors and good advice they offer. To the largely unacknowledged and often taken-for-granted experts who constitute the world of medical education.

Who Are the Invisible Workers of Medical Education?

One of the most challenging elements of compiling this volume is the fact that we could never do justice to the diversity of people, backgrounds, skill sets, roles, and expertise we find in any given medical school or academic teaching hospital. As soon as it seemed we had arrived at a relatively fulsome list of workers and jobs to include, we would realize that we'd missed someone essential and important – and in overlooking that role, we were reproducing the very invisibilities we were seeking to undo. And for that, we apologize. The chapters that follow only describe some of the people, the variety of roles, and the striking creativity and energy people bring to their work in our field.

One of the best ways to identify the multiple invisible workers, and the invisible work that they do, is to work with an illustration. Returning to our earlier, familiar example of a lecture, let's begin with a question: what is the work associated with delivering a lecture?

You would most likely turn your attention to the professor. We picture the professor – likely invited to teach on the topic because they hold specialized knowledge – who prepares the content, makes a deck of PowerPoint slides, and arrives in a classroom to teach. They stand in front of the room and speak to each slide, weaving together knowledge and experience while students sit attentively, listening and taking notes.

But, when we consider the lecture from the standpoint of unravelling the layers of work involved, and the (in)visibility of each of those layers, the complexity of all of our tasks, even one as familiar as a lecture, becomes apparent.

First of all, with respect to *education delivery*, the lecture is part of a broader curriculum. At some point, a group of people came together to coherently schedule a curriculum of educational activities addressing all the essential knowledge, skills, and attitudes a medical student must hold at graduation to be competent to move onto graduate training. A group of administrators within the medical school must have worked to ensure that students are receiving instruction in these various essential skills. People decided when each lecture would be delivered and the amount of time allotted to each lecture. Someone decided which topics were amenable to a lecture as opposed to those that needed some hands-on procedural skill instruction, for example. Someone broke the topic down into accomplishable learning objectives to be met via the lecture, and someone mapped those objectives up to the broader expected outcomes of the curriculum. People interviewed, hired, and paid the best teachers to deliver the lecture. In sum, just to deliver one lecture, a veritable army of people were needed to realize the delivery of the educational session.

From the perspective of *evidence assembly*, the content of the lecture had to come from somewhere. Somewhere along the way, a researcher worked with someone from their institution to plan a research proposal. Someone from library staff may have worked with the researcher to make sure their proposal was complete with the most up-to-date evidence. The successful research grant had to be coordinated with someone who works in the finance office and ethics offices to ensure that funds would be responsibly handled and that participants could be responsibly recruited. Research assistants and graduate students likely contributed to the project, hopefully helping to turn findings into actionable information, which eventually found its way into print. All of this, and even more invisible work, had to happen well before our lecturer could stand in front of a group of students to deliver the content.

With respect to *institutional concerns*, someone had to ensure that the lecture was physically accessible and structurally possible. Someone attended to the significant task of guaranteeing that learners could physically access the lecture room, and that the technology required to see and hear the lecture was functioning. Some ensured that the learners knew about the lecture and that it was listed in learners' formal calendars. Someone made sure faculty members were prepared to teach, and someone else helped to ensure that the content was consistent with required accreditation standards. And, hopefully, a number of people were on board to support diverse learners and faculty to be valued and appreciated. And somebody made sure the heat was on in the winter and the air conditioning was running in the summer. Together, with many other invisible workers, these people ensured that the institution was running so that the lecture could happen.

In the world of medical education, many of the jobs and tasks we've described above are familiar to us, but they happen backstage and remain largely unacknowledged. However, regardless of how much we know about these jobs, we all know that within each role there are things that must be done that escape any sort of formal classification. These subtleties – everything from sweet-talking challenging personalities, to knowing who to call when things go wrong, to offering support in the form of a listening ear or words of kindness – are largely unacknowledged and unremunerated. The development of such a body of expertise is crucial; however, this type of work falls outside of the ways in which we traditionally think about work. And so, while we all appreciate it, we rarely pause to think about it.

Exploring Invisible Work in This Volume

In this edited collection, we've convened an international group of celebrated scholars of medical education, clinicians, and practitioners to come together to acknowledge the cast of thousands involved with medical education and to contextualize the invaluable contributions made by these people. Our goal is to recognize and explain why those skills and talents are essential to the education of physicians; we also will question why these contributions are largely overlooked.

What makes this volume unique and, we believe, important, is that we've invited the people who do these invisible jobs to tell their stories in their own words. Each chapter is written by a team of authors, one of whom falls into the category of an invisible worker. And in each chapter we've chosen to centre the stories of these workers to broaden the width of the spotlight and highlight their savvy and their essential status.

The volume is divided into three broad categories of work related to medical education: 1. Education Delivery, 2. Evidence Assembly, and 3. Institutional Concerns. Each section begins with a framing chapter that provides background information and reflections about the invisible work addressed in the chapters of the category.

Within the Education Delivery section, we turn the spotlight to some of the less well-known workers involved with medical teaching. Moving beyond the image of a professor in front of a lecture theatre, we'll explore some of the other types of labour involved with medical education, including making decisions about admissions (Chapter 6), preparing educational materials, like anatomical pro-sections and cadavers (Chapter 3), and supporting anxious students through an assessment (Chapter 5). We'll also highlight some of the specialized skills people bring to the enterprise of medical education from a variety of different backgrounds and professions, including acting (Chapter 4), funeral directing (Chapter 3), Licensed Practical Nursing (Chapter 8), and social work (Chapter 7).

In the Evidence Assembly section, we'll investigate the work involved with translating medical education research and scholarship into practice. We'll explore the use of data and application of theory in program evaluation (Chapter 10). We'll turn to poetry to express the complexity of the graduate student experience (Chapter 11). We'll investigate the invisible expertise associated with fostering relationships when it comes to preparing research grants (Chapter 14), planning conferences (Chapter 13), and supporting research assistants (Chapter 11).

In the section addressing Institutional Concerns, we'll learn about the complexity of equity, diversity, and inclusion work in medical schools (Chapter 16), and think about the emotionally challenging work of learning medicine (Chapter 21). We'll unpack the catch-all term "technology" and learn about the various roles and areas of expertise at work behind the scenes in any given Information Technology (IT) department (Chapter 17). We'll shine a light on the tremendous expertise needed behind the scenes as people juggle competing priorities of the workplace settings (Chapter 20) and manage any unexpected situation that will need to be managed (Chapter 18). And we'll illuminate the social and global phenomenon of accreditation (Chapter 19).

The complexity of medical education – its tasks, its goals, and its people – make it a beautifully complex and constantly evolving thing. Traditionally, medical education as a discipline has emphasized the work involved in teaching and learning content knowledge, professional attitudes, and technical skills, but the critical role of the invisible work that supports it all, everything from research to clinical practice, cannot be overstated.

We believe turning our attention to the invisible work of medical education may help us to think (differently, or even at all) about the essentialness of administrative work, emotional labour, and support work that happens at every medical school around the world, as our international team of authors can attest. And while we certainly offer this volume as a spotlight for highlighting the multiple talents of the people in our community, we also hope that these chapters serve to reaffirm for medical learners, no matter where they sit on the educational continuum, the complexity of medical education, medicine, and healthcare systems. Certainly, *all* members of our community have a valuable role to play and a meaningful story to tell.

And so, we invite you to make space in your heart *and* mind as you read through the chapters that follow. Listen carefully to the songs sung by this chorus of unheard voices. Once you've heard them, we hope their stories and their work will no longer be invisible. Perhaps, once you've heard them, you too can help to ensure that the skills, expertise, and essential value of these individuals is acknowledged and rewarded.

References

1. Watson, T.J. 1995. *Sociology, Work and Industry*, 3rd edn. Routledge.
2. Morris, C. 2018. Work-Based Learning. In *Understanding Medical Education*, edited by T. Swanwick, K. Forrest, and B.C. O'Brien, 163–77. https://doi.org/10.1002/9781119373780.ch12
3. Dornan, T., Boshuizen, H., King, N., and Scherpbier, A. 2007. Experience-based learning: a model linking the processes and outcomes of medical students' workplace learning. *Medical Education*, 41(1), 84–91. https://doi.org/10.1111/j.1365-2929.2006.02652.x
4. Swanwick, T. 2005. Informal learning in postgraduate medical education: from cognitivism to "culturism". *Medical Education*, 39(8), 859–65. https://doi.org/10.1111/j.1365-2929.2005.02224.x

5. Ayala-Hurtado, E., and Lamont, M. 2021. Sociology of work meets cultural sociology: Thoughts on Arne Kalleberg's *Precarious Lives: Job insecurity and Well-Being in Rich Democracies. Contemporary Sociology*, 50(2), 111–14. https://doi.org/10.1177/0094306121991073c

6. Wharton, A.S. 2009. The sociology of emotional labor. *Annual Review of Sociology*, 35(1), 147–65. https://doi.org/10.1146/annurev-soc-070308-115944

7. Kalleberg, A.L. 2009. Precarious work, insecure workers: Employment relations in transition. *American Sociological Review*, 74(1), 1–22. https://doi.org/10.1177/000312240907400101

8. Gopal, R., Glasheen, J.J., Miyoshi, T.J., and Prochazka, A.V. 2005. Burnout and internal medicine resident work-hour restrictions. *Archives of Internal Medicine*, 165(22), 2595–600. https://doi.org/10.1001/archinte.165.22.2595

9. Jephson, N., Cook, H., and Charlwood, A. 2023. Prisoners of oath: Junior doctors' professional identities during and after industrial action. *Economic and Industrial Democracy*, 45(2), 556–78. https://doi.org/10.1177/0143831X231175701

10. Ranasinghe, P.D. 2015. International medical graduates in the US physician workforce. *Journal of Osteopathic Medicine*, 115(4), 236–41. https://doi.org/10.7556/jaoa.2015.047

11. Garavand, A., Jalali, S., Talebi, A.H., and Sabahi, A. 2022. Advantages and disadvantages of teleworking in healthcare institutions during COVID-19: A systematic review. *Informatics in Medicine Unlocked*, 34, 101119. https://doi.org/10.1016/j.imu.2022.101119

12. Shah, D.T., Williams, V.N., Thorndyke, L.E., Marsh, E.E., Sonnino, R.E., Block, S.M., and Viggiano, T.R. 2018. Restoring faculty vitality in academic medicine when burnout threatens. *Academic Medicine*, 93(7), 979. https://doi.org/10.1097/ACM.0000000000002013

13. Merton, R.K. 1934. Durkheim's division of labor in society. *American Journal of Sociology*, 40(3):319–28. http://www.jstor.org/stable/2768264

14. Treiman, D.J. 1970. Industrialization and social stratification. *Sociological Inquiry*, 40(2), 207–34. https://doi.org/10.1111/j.1475-682X.1970.tb01009.x

15. Star, S.L. and Strauss, A. 1999. Layers of silence, arenas of voice: the ecology of visible and invisible work. *Computer Supported Cooperative Work (CSCW)*, 8, 9–30. https://doi.org/10.1023/A:1008651105359

16. Goffman, E. 1959. *The Presentation of Self in Everyday Life*. Anchor Books.

17. Vinson, A.H. and Underman, K. 2020. Clinical empathy as emotional labor in medical work. *Social Science & Medicine*, 251, 112904.

18. Abdellatif, W., Ding, J., Jalal, S., Chopra, S., Butler, J., Ali, I.T., Shah, S., and Khosa, F. 2019. Leadership gender disparity within research-intensive medical schools: a transcontinental thematic analysis. *Journal of Continuing Education in the Health Professions*, 39(4), 243–50. https://doi.org/10.1097/CEH.0000000000000270

19. Marmot, M. and Allen, J.J. 2014. Social determinants of health equity. *American Journal of Public Health*, 104(S4), S517–19. https://doi.org/10.2105/AJPH.2014.302200

20. He, J.C., Kang, S.K., Tse, K., and Toh, S.M. 2019. Stereotypes at work: occupational stereotypes predict race and gender segregation in the workforce. *Journal of Vocational Behavior*, 115, 103318. https://doi.org/10.1016/j.jvb.2019.103318

21. Crites, S.N., Dickson, K.E., and Lorenz, A. 2015. Nurturing gender stereotypes in the face of experience: a study of leader gender, leadership style, and satisfaction. *Journal of Organizational Culture, Communications and Conflict*, 19(1), 1.

22. Azzarito, L. 2019. *Social Justice in Globalized Fitness and Health: Bodies Out of Sight*. Routledge.

23. Colliver, J.A., Swartz, M.H., and Robbs, R.S. 2001, The effect of examinee and patient ethnicity in clinical-skills assessment with standardized patients. *Advances in Health Sciences Education*, 6, 5–13. https://doi.org/10.1023/a:1009864529376

24. Yu, P.T., Parsa, P.V., Hassanein, O., Rogers, S.O., and Chang, D.C. 2013. Minorities struggle to advance in academic medicine: a 12-y review of diversity at the highest levels of America's teaching institutions. *Journal of Surgical Research*, 182(2) 212–18. https://doi.org/10.1016/j.jss.2012.06.049

25. Campbell, K.M. and Rodríguez, J.E. 2019. Addressing the minority tax: perspectives from two diversity leaders on building minority faculty success in academic medicine. *Academic Medicine*, 94(12), 1854–7. https://doi.org/10.1097/ACM.0000000000002839

26. Bhatt, W. 2013. The little brown woman: gender discrimination in American medicine. *Gender & Society*, 27(5), 659–80. https://doi.org/10.1177/0891243213491140

27. Crain, M., Poster, W., and Cherry, M., eds. 2016. *Invisible Labor: Hidden Work in the Contemporary World*. University of California Press.

28. Xiaoming, Y., Ma, B.J., Chang, C.L., and Shieh, C.J. 2014. Effects of workload on burnout and turnover intention of medical staff: a study. *Studies on Ethno-medicine*, 8(3), 229–37. https://doi.org/10.31901/24566772.2014/08.03.04

PART ONE

Education Delivery

2 Education Delivery – Framing Chapter: Us and Them

RACHEL H. ELLAWAY

Us and them, and after all, we're only ordinary men.

"Us and Them" by Pink Floyd, 1973

In writing this chapter, I was reminded again and again of the song "Us and Them" on Pink Floyd's Dark Side of the Moon album, which explores difference and exclusion and its consequences. It is in considering "us and them" that I start this chapter. Separating the world into us and them is a primitive reaction that reinforces the "us" of family and tribe while making enemies of everyone else as "them." This has been extensively theorized as "in group" and "out group" behaviour.[1] However, rather than saying "them" in respect of invisible workers, maybe I should say "us," as medical education researchers (who constitute many of the authors of this volume) can arguably be understood both as insiders and outsiders. Researchers may be visible (perhaps even hypervisible) in terms of research products (papers, books, presentations) and through other recognitions (awards, appointments), but they may not be seen to be fully part of the educational enterprise unless they participate in other roles (as teachers, administrators, developers, etc.). Indeed, as in H.G. Wells' dystopic vision of the future of mankind, to some they may seem like the superficial Eloi compared to the Morlocks doing the actual work of health professions education (HPE).[2] Of course, the Morlocks were portrayed as less than ideal role models, not least in their dietary choices.

I should also say "us" as, in my time, I have worked in medical illustration, been an educational technologist and an instructional designer, and been an administrator, all in the service of medical education. Indeed, despite my time as an education researcher, it sometimes seems that I have never left those other worlds. I know first-hand the wonderful experiences and opportunities that such roles can afford, I know too the sense of exclusion and second-class status that such roles can bring. It was not my plan to be a medical educator. To be honest, I am still not sure what I want to be when I grow up. Maybe we should seek, or at least try to embrace, degrees of invisibility. Maybe we are all partly invisible but we never noticed.

Invisible People

What does invisibility mean as a construct applied to those who work in medical education? Is someone invisible because they cannot be seen or because they have simply evaded notice? Is someone invisible because they have been deliberately treated as such, or have they faded from view through overfamiliarity or the disinterest of others? Is the person invisible to some but not others? Is the person invisible even to themselves? What might render a person visible again and with what consequences? These are questions underpinning the core theses of this volume, first that there are many individuals who work in medical education who are treated as if they were invisible, and second that this invisibility should be challenged and explored.

This is not simply an academic exercise. To be invisible as a person has long been associated with social constructs of class, caste, and social hierarchy. Invisible workers may be like Gramsci's subalterns, a group central to the functioning of a colonial organization but excluded from any power. Invisible workers may be like Roald Dahl's Oompa Loompas, a people acting as a (supposedly) willing underclass.[3] Invisible workers may be like servants in grand houses who are seen but not heard, working "below stairs" in spaces that are adjacent to but distinct from the spaces of those they serve. None of these framings is particularly positive or empowering, nor do they reflect the rich and honourable contributions invisible workers can make to an enterprise. The word "invisible" hangs there, potent and troubling in its implications. A less problematic reading of invisible workers reflects a similar issue to that of the hidden curriculum, in that these workers fulfil intentional and important roles but are functionally tacit rather than socially elided. We should ask too whether there is a meaningful difference between these perspectives. Even where there is no intentional oppression or control, hierarchies and divisions of labour, authority and legitimacy can create them.

Troubling Invisibility

Who, then, is invisible in medical education? A faculty originally referred plurally to its scholars rather than to the institution, and as such we might argue that the professoriate is intrinsically visible. However, with the growing corporatization of post-secondary institutions and the dominance of neoliberal thinking and culture, this is less and less the case.[4] If post-secondary educational institutions (PSEIs) are becoming more corporate in their cultures and functions, then surely their leaders and managers are visible for their authority and role in "making things happen." Yes, they can be "seen," but they too can become somewhat invisible outside of their rounds of meetings and grand offices. Models of bicameral governance (separating corporate and academic governance processes) are commonly found in most PSEIs, meaning that academics are largely invisible in corporate governance, and vice versa. Moreover, much teaching is undertaken by adjunct professors and other individuals with little ability to be seen or treated as a part of the professoriate. In medical education these can include standardized patient educators and anatomy demonstrators. Invisibility, rather than being a binary matter of being "in" or "out," might be better understood as a matter of authority and responsibility; the less one has the less visible one becomes.

What about the students? Surely they are visible? They are, after all, the primary focus of medical education. Students can certainly have visibility as a collective (a class, a cohort), but they tend to be far less visible as individuals. Indeed, much of the hidden curriculum is about obedience and compliance, not just with program rules and regulations, but with the tacit culture of the profession they seek to join. I could argue, therefore, that students' visibility as a whole is decreased in medical training by their assimilation of its identities and norms. There is also the question of those students who actively seek invisibility, whether from introversion or more worryingly as a way of concealing their shortcomings. It is interesting to observe from this that invisibility may be sought as well as conferred. Indeed, I would argue that invisibility is not just a challenging construct for the professions reflected in this volume; it is troubling for all medical education.

So what does invisibility mean? These individuals are clearly not transparent or visible only to ultraviolet or X-ray radiation. Indeed, many of them are paid employees and so have contracts, workplaces, and material recognition for their contributions. Even those volunteering their labour (such as admissions file reviewers) are typically acknowledged in some other way. When we talk of invisibility in medical education, I would argue we mean (albeit variably) three specific things. First, we may be referring to invisibility in the discourses and representations of medical education, such as research papers, presentations, and websites. The invisible people of medical education are like ghosts in these spaces, occasionally mentioned but largely not, mostly implied in the descriptions of medical education activities and programs. Second, we may be referring to invisibility in the governance and direction of medical education, which comes down to legitimacy and authority. Even if an erstwhile invisible person participates in governance, it is usually in ways circumscribed by their immediate role. Third, we may be referring to invisibility from a particular perspective, typically our own. This is a peep-bo/peekaboo kind of invisibility: if I cannot see something, then I will treat it as if it does not exist. Someone who is invisible to me may be visible to others, and vice versa. This suggests that invisibility is a relative concept and in great part depends on the observer (and their authority) rather than on the observed. Clearly, invisibility is more than a condition of a role or person; it is a systemic construct that reflects many underlying structures and assumptions of medical education as a whole.

Economics of Invisibility

Although it is often not acknowledged in academic discourses, economic factors are the primary drivers of what is and is not actually done in medical education. Educational theory and research may suggest many kinds of good and effective practices, but what from this body of knowledge is taken up depends on resources and other necessary constraints and compromises educators face.[5] Is invisibility something we might understand from an economic perspective? I would argue that many of the invisible roles explored in this book attract lower salaries than faculty members and administrators; they tend to be in different unions; and they have different rights. Many of them are treated as workers rather than as academics and are seen as having jobs rather than careers.

We might take a critical neoliberal perspective on these arrangements, exploring constructions of invisible work in terms of paying lower salaries to those with less bargaining power to do the work that otherwise might be done by academics. On the other hand, we might argue that academics should do academic work and technical work should be done by technicians. So how does the distribution of labour in medical education spaces work? How are lines of demarcation set up by contracts and collective agreements, and how are these lines crossed or blurred? Where, if anywhere, should the division of labour be? Is it about skills, ability, and competence or about organizational control? Are invisible workers in medical education, like the growing use of sessional instructors in much of higher education, a reflection of economic rather than academic policy?

I have seen many situations where academics were doing the work of invisible workers, and many where invisible workers were doing the work of academics. Clearly there is no hard-and-fast demarcation between the two; rather, there are organizational accommodations about where these boundaries lie and how they are policed. Risk and obedience are also part of this equation. Academic freedom and the entrepreneurial aspects of being a part of the professoriate afford a lot of latitude in what we do. Most of the invisible workers in medical education have a lot less autonomy. From this, we might explore issues of agency, autonomy, and discretion in how invisible workers do what they do. For instance, invisible workers may express dissatisfaction and dissent by slowing down or working to rule. Indeed, they may have many ways of engaging with the medical education systems that are not available or meaningful to academics, who have a shared responsibility in the processes and outcomes of academic programming. Having said that, I know of many invisible workers who are committed to education scholarship, and many dissatisfied scholars who lack the commitment shown by their invisible colleagues.

Legitimate Participation

While faculty and student roles are deeply embedded in the fabric of post-secondary institutions, support roles tend to be relatively new and less grounded in academic cultures. We should ask, therefore: what are the shared identities and cultures of professions such as these? Can we even consider them to be professions in the same way as we think of healthcare professionals or the professoriate? From a personal perspective, I have known and employed many invisible workers. Some of them wanted to pursue academic careers and therefore aligned themselves with the academic mission. Some of them were creatives or other kinds of professionals who had a professional identity outside of academe (such as programmers, multimedia artists, graphic designers, and illustrators).

Legitimacy is not just a matter of whether or to what degree someone belongs in medical education; it can reflect a sense of being a legitimate participant in other professions. For programmers, administrators, lawyers, and others for whom there are well-established professional bodies and recognition, legitimacy need not come from within medical education. Indeed, those invisible workers with a strong professional identity outside the academy may see themselves more like specialists whose professional culture is that of their specialty rather than the organization who engages their services. On the other hand, demonstrators, simulated patients, instructional designers, non-academic statisticians, and others who sit much closer to academic practice may have a harder time establishing an identity outside the sphere of medical education. A lot comes down to what one's community of practice is and with whom it is shared. It might be that the most invisible workers are those who fall between the cracks; they have no professional identity outside of medical education and yet are invisible within it. Not all invisibility is the same. Some kinds can be much more isolating than others.

A Changing Landscape

Faculty and students have power and relational structures with roots in the deep past, and as such they sit at the very heart of the academic institution and the academic enterprise. Many invisible workers' roles, on the other hand, are relatively new, and they sit uneasily within an academic framework. Many of these roles (such as those in information technology [IT]) have sprung into existence only within a generation or so, while more well-established roles such as anatomy instructors or medical illustrators have more depth within the academy, albeit one that has diminished over time. Indeed, while the details of faculty, students, and leadership roles change, they have persisted for centuries. The roles of invisible workers, however, come and go according to the changing winds and expectations of medical education practice. This in turn could weaken invisible workers' sense of belonging or participation in medical education as an enterprise. Indeed, invisibility may also have connotations of disposability and uncertainty.

Changing trends in HPE can also impact visibility in terms of to what extent invisible workers are woven into its narratives and discourses. Some of these roles have been researched and evaluated a lot more than others. Standardized patients, for instance, have been researched rather more than test administrators and statisticians have, at least as far as reviews of the literature have indicated.[6,7] Invisibility, from this perspective, might be equated with fashions and the collective interest and attention of medical education scholars. That is not to say there are not systemic elisions or biases. For instance, there are few, if any, national or international newspapers or magazines for medical education, nor are there any dedicated news channels or other media outlets to communicate what is happening in medical education. The narratives of medical education are primarily articulated through academic journals, institutional websites, and social media. Invisibility may also be a product of a gap in the kinds of stories we tell and the places that such stories can be told.

In This Section

This section considers a number of perspectives of those involved in different areas of invisible work in medical education. In Chapter 3, Luong et al. describe the invisible work of those running clinical cadaver programs in medical education. Although the technical work in handling and preparing bodies for instructional use is carried out in private spaces and is thus out of sight, it is visible in the sense that this work is acknowledged by others. However, other aspects of their role are more invisible in that they are often not even guessed at, such as facilitating body donation through working with the families of the deceased, or organizing ceremonies to celebrate the lives of the donors. Luong et al. also raise the issue of social stigma associated with dissection and death as a contributing factor to their invisibility.

In Chapter 4, Lynée et al. describe the invisible work of simulated patients in medical education. While they are not invisible to the learners who interact with them, the influence of simulated patients in medical education as a whole is limited. It is also interesting to see that simulated patients do not simply turn up, do their thing, and leave. They are often involved in case writing, in advancing the underlying educational goals of particular interactions, and in helping all actors to reflect on what is being portrayed and how. This depth and off-camera activity is their invisible work, as is their bringing lay perspectives to bear on otherwise institutionalized constructions of patient encounters.

In Chapter 5, Ryan et al. describe many new and divergent roles and responsibilities that have been brought about by innovations in assessment, both technological and procedural. New processes require different skills and responsibilities, and they create different dependencies and complexities. Interestingly, although the subjects considered themselves largely invisible to their stakeholders, the functional invisibility of their roles was considered an indication of effectiveness in carrying out these roles.

In Chapter 6, Burm et al. describe administrative roles within the context of medical school admissions, arguing that, since who is allowed in is one of the most important factors in the success (or otherwise) of medical education, the products of that work are at the very heart of medical education, even though their contribution may be invisible to many. There is a social calling to this work as well as one of performing consistently at a high standard and often under some duress.

In Chapter 7, Hoffman et al. describe the work of community and community healthcare providers in medical education. As more attention has been given to education outside of academic health science centres, the liaison between schools and community partners has become a critical part of medical training. However, this work is, as they say, "complex and messy," not least because practice environments and cultures outside of academic health science centres is also invisible to those within them. As with those working in admissions, there is a moral dimension to this work, particularly in seeking to address systemic inequities and invisibilities within healthcare as a whole.

Systemic equity issues are also explored in Chapter 8, where Olmos-Vega et al. describe the work of Licensed Practice Nurses in learning about interprofessional care. Invisibility here is twofold – the presence and legitimacy of nurses teaching future doctors about interprofessional care and collaboration, and the authority they have in doing so. This underscores the power wielded by medical hierarchies to render whole health professional groups relatively invisible.

Concluding Thoughts

There are many issues covered in the coming chapters that I encourage you, dear reader, to reflect on. These include varying degrees of invisibility, the social construction of invisibility, invisibility as a positive thing, the transference of invisibility from healthcare as a whole to medical education, the need to work past invisibility if things are ever to change, and the invisibility of the dependence of medical education on so many of these roles.

Although the idea of "invisible workers" might seem to suggest their complicity as well as our own (writing as a medical education scholar) in their elision from the discourses of medical education, the following chapters challenge this in so many ways. Clearly, we need to understand education systems in ways that include those who do not fit into the traditional narratives of the professoriate and their students. Welcome to the "long tail" of contemporary medical education.

References

1. Tajfel, H. 1970. Experiments in intergroup discrimination. *Scientific American*, 223(5), 96–102. https://doi.org/10.1038/scientificamerican1170-96
2. Wells, H.G. (1895). *The Time Machine*. Heinemann.
3. Dahl, R. 1964. *Charlie and the Chocolate Factory*. Knopf.
4. Staller, K.M. 2022. Beware the kudzu: corporate creep, university consumers, and epistemic injustice. *Qualitative Social Work*, 21(4), 643–59. https://doi.org/10.1177/14733250221106639

5. Thomas, A. and Ellaway, R.H. 2021. Rethinking implementation science for health professional education: a manifesto for change. *Perspectives on Medical Education*, 10(6), 362–8. https://doi.org/10.1007/s40037-021-00688-3

6. May, W., Park, J.H., and Lee, J.P. 2009. A ten-year review of the literature on the use of standardized patients in teaching and learning: 1996–2005. *Medical Teacher*, 31(6), 487–92. https://doi.org/10.1080/01421590802530898

7. Wilbur, K., Elmubark, A. and Shabana, S. 2018. Systematic review of standardized patient use in continuing medical education. *Journal of Continuing Education in the Health Professions*, 38(1), 3–10. https://doi.org/10.1097/CEH.0000000000000190

3 Voices from the Underground: Cadaver Work and Medical Education

VICTORIA LUONG, GEORGE KOVACS, ROBERT SANDESKI, AND ANNA MACLEOD

Every year, before classes start, we have the students gather around the cadaver and we – usually a faculty member and myself – will have an open conversation with them. We'll ask, maybe, who has experienced death and how that death relates to them. Many having never experienced death ... to stand at the foot of a cadaver can be a little over-whelming. Last year, there was one medical student who I could tell was really strug-gling. So, as the students started to disperse, I had a chance to go over and talk to her. She said, "I've never dealt with death before." And in medical school, once your feet hit the ground, there's no looking back ... so, she was worried that she was going to fall behind because of that. But, over the next couple of days before lab started, I invited her back, and we eased into it, gradually exposing the hand, a little bit of the arm, until we got to the point where she felt comfortable. At the time, it didn't mean much for me – it was just another day. But it meant a lot to her, and she has come back to talk to me every time I see her. And she'll tell me, "I would have never got through Med school if it wasn't for your kindness." Those experiences come up quite often. That human con-nection that we have to be able to grapple with.

Rob Sandeski

When we talk about cadaver work in medical education, what imme-diately comes to mind? We might think of the medical student who is experiencing, for the first time, the coldness of the body, the smell of the embalming fluid, the sterility of the surgical table, or the mixed feelings of shock and awe that arise when coming face to face with a dead body. We might think of the teacher, who is using the cadaver as a tool for demon-strating the intricate anatomical details of the human body, who is show-ing their students how to manoeuvre the cadaver in just the right way, or who educates them about the importance of paying respect to the donor.

But when do we think about the people involved behind the scenes in cadaver-based education? We know that these bodies have been donated – but how did these bodies find themselves in a simulation suite, cleaned, draped, and ready to be dissected? Who ensures that the process of procuring, using, and returning the bodies to their families is conducted efficiently and humanely? How is it that we have the privilege of learning with these bodies in the first place?

In this chapter, we will explore the invisible work of clinical cadaver programs – i.e., the programs that manage the procurement, preparation, and return of the human bodies for education of undergraduate, graduate, and continuing medical learners around the world. Specifically, we address the Dalhousie University Human Body Donation Program (HBD), which supports the use of approximately 170 bodies a year from across Maritime Canada for use in anatomy labs and procedural skill teaching. The HBD works closely with the Clinical Cadaver Program (CCP) to provide newly deceased, previously frozen, soft-preserved cadavers for teaching medical students, residents, and practising physicians in multiple educational programs. Although we rarely stop to think about what the people involved in these programs do in their day-to-day work, their practices are essential to trainees' experiences with this precious educational resource.

Cadaver-Based Medical Education: An Academic Perspective

Cadavers have been used to study human anatomy for over 2,000 years. Due to ever-evolving ideas about the sanctity of the human body, the history of its adoption as a teaching tool for medical students has been far from straightforward.[1,2] However, since the Anatomy Act – which outlined the legal and procedural details required for ethical body procurement and dissection in Nova Scotia, Canada – was established in 1832, cadaveric dissection has evolved into what is now a mainstay of medical education in most of the world.[3–5]

Although cadavers have traditionally been used as anatomical models, the utility of cadavers for medical education is changing. With the modernization of techniques for preservation and embalming, it is now possible to prepare cadavers that resemble living, anesthetized patients with strikingly high degrees of fidelity.[6,7] Instead of using formaldehyde as the primary fixative, these realistic cadavers are prepared using a mixture of chemicals that better retain the colour, elasticity, and consistency of living tissue.[6,8] Because they maintain the look and feel of living patients, these soft-preserved cadavers can be used not only to study the anatomical structure of the human body, but also to practise rare and often life-saving procedures like hepatectomies,[9] vascular trauma surgery,[10] and laparoscopic liver surgery.[11] At Dalhousie Medical

School, these cadavers are called *clinical cadavers* and are regularly used in cadaver-based simulation (CBS) to teach medical students, residents, and practising physicians procedures such as emergency intubation, thoracotomies, and lateral canthotomies.

As both teachers and learners can attest, no model of the human body can simulate a real patient like a cadaver.[12–14] Compared to plastic manikins, the cadaver shows more realistic responses to touch, like jaw mobility and neck flexibility,[15] lung inflation during bag-mask ventilation,[6] and functional obstructions during an attempted laryngoscopy.[6] In addition, while manikins are designed to be representative of the "standard" patient – as if there were such a thing – cadavers show the variability in body composition that students will encounter in real life.[16] Moreover, cadavers are essential not only because of how accurately they depict human anatomy, but also because of what they are: human.[17] Gunderman and Wilson[18] liken the experience of working with cadavers to when the host of a dinner party mentions some distant land:

> They ... can call to mind not only photographs of the place from a book but who has actually trodden the ground, felt the climate, and touched the people. Whether it is the heart, the lungs, the liver, the brain, or the joints, the medical student who has actually participated in cadaver dissection can say not only, "I know what that looks like," but also "I have been there." (p. 746)

In a 2022 paper,[14] we argued that the *ontological fidelity* of the cadaver is what makes it a truly irreplaceable resource for medical education. Ontology refers to the study of being (what something is); a cadaver has something beyond what the most cutting-edge manikin will ever be able to simulate: it is human. And the humanness of the cadaver makes students learn in a distinctly unique way; that is, with the level engagement, compassion, and respect that the donors deserve. In this way, students not only learn about the technical aspects of their training, but also about the moral landscape within which they are practising.

Research on cadaver-based medical education has previously explored the potential uses of cadavers for anatomical education[4] and procedural skills,[6] and tested their efficacy compared to other educational models.[15,19] Scholars in the field have traced the complicated history of the use of cadavers,[2] including the evolution of human body donation.[20] Many have debated the necessity of cadaver work, particularly in the post-COVID era of technological innovation.[21] Others have documented the experience of medical students navigating cadaveric dissection,[22] the various physical and emotional reactions they might have to them,[23] and the importance of cadavers for teaching empathy and morality.[24,25]

Despite such growing recognition of the importance of cadavers in the education of medical learners, however, there has been little attention paid to the actual work that needs to occur for cadaver-based education to be carried out day-to-day. The roles and responsibilities of those involved have long been overlooked, even though cadaver-based pedagogy would not exist without them. These people include, for example:

1. Managers, who oversee the entire program and work closely with the families of donors;
2. Administrators, who maintain records, assist with scheduling and planning, and help develop program material;
3. Technicians, who embalm, prepare, and maintain the cadavers;
4. Inspectors, who receive and record every death in the province and monitor the program to ensure compliance to acts and policies;
5. Teachers and teaching assistants, who develop curriculum material and teach anatomy/procedural skills with cadavers;
6. Transportation staff, who move cadavers between various locations; and
7. Clergy, who speak at the interment and memorial services.

To illustrate the invisible work of a clinical cadaver program, we highlight two perspectives: George Kovacs, Emergency Physician and Medical Director, Clinical Cadaver Program, who addresses the importance of having advocates for educational innovations; and Robert Sandeski, Manager of the Human Body Donation Program, who highlights the overlapping technical, organizational, and relational aspects that are necessary to cadaver work.

Cadaver-Based Medical Education: A Physician's Perspective

Around 2000, I was working with a colleague on developing an airway management device. One of the challenges with airway devices – or any device – is how to train students to transition from practising with a plastic manikin to using them on a real person. At the time, my colleague and friend, Richard Levitan, who shared my interest in airway management, was offering opportunities to work with soft-preserved cadavers in Baltimore. So, I asked Richard if my colleague and I could come down to try our device on their cadavers.

We flew down, with a couple suitcases of equipment, and went to the basement of this old building in Baltimore. We started to work, and within about

20 minutes, we were just blown away. These cadavers were incredibly realistic, and we were using one after another. We left there forgetting about our device and talking about what an educational tool this could be.

We flew back. And, the next morning, I looked up where the anatomy offices were, walked up, knocked on the door, and asked to speak to the department head. I said, listen, you and Rob Sandeski (the lead technician at the time) need to go to Baltimore. I'll help you with funding ... You just need to go. Within a week after they returned, they had prepared the first cadaver using the technique from Baltimore.

Things progressed from there, but the real turning point for the cadaver program was when we converted a garage into a trauma bay and staged a simulation for the residents on call. On that day, just like what happens in real life, the residents who were acting as trauma team leaders were paged into the resuscitation room, and then into the trauma bay, where all the equipment – and even nurses – were waiting for them. A real ambulance showed up, bringing out a cadaver, on which they had to open up the chest and insert a breathing tube. The dean witnessed all of this, was blown away, and that was the trigger for us to receive funding to convert it into what is now a $1.5 million simulation bay.

Since we started the program, we have expanded from taking in one to about 170 cadavers a year. We were accredited with special commendation by the Royal College because of the CCP. We received recognition in terms of quality awards and research publications. And, importantly, Rob Sandeski received a leadership role in the HBD program, which was a critical acknowledgment of the importance of the work that he does.

– George Kovacs, Medical Director, Clinical Cadaver Program

When educational opportunities are presented to us, it's easy to forget that – at one point in time – the learning activity had to be developed and implemented. And perhaps more importantly, we easily forget that this "opportunity" had to be developed and implemented *by someone.* It takes someone (or a group of people) to recognize a gap in our educational practices, to seek out innovations that can address that gap, and to assemble resources to plan and implement a solution.

The amount of work involved in establishing and maintaining a clinical cadaver program cannot be overstated. Procuring deceased human bodies for the purposes of education is both ethically and logistically complex. As noted above, a human donation program needs access to donors, in addition to a number of skilled workers for procuring, preparing, maintaining, and transporting bodies. It needs appropriate facilities for education and storage, and financial resources to accomplish all of these tasks. Due to the sensitive nature of this work, all of the operations of the HBD program must adhere to the Cemeteries Act, the Fatalities Act, the Funeral Directors and Embalmers Act, and the Anatomy Act of Nova Scotia.

Without resourceful and dedicated people to do the work of finding solutions to multiple organizational, financial, and political barriers, much of the educational opportunities that have become part of our day-to-day practices would not exist. The individuals who work in cadaver-based education are instrumental to the education of skilled physicians. Without these people – who do all their work hidden away in basements of medical education facilities everywhere – our physicians would not be the competent practitioners that they are today.

Cadaver-Based Medical Education: A Technician's Perspective

There are so many different aspects to my job that it's hard to put into a paragraph or two. On one level, my job involves managing the intake of bodies. I'm essentially on call 24/7, 7 days a week, 365 days a year, because when a donor dies … that needs to be dealt with immediately. Then, my job also involves cadaver care. I work with two other technicians, both licensed funeral directors, who help with all the prep work, cadaver maintenance, and the day-to-day set-up and tear-down of the labs.

– Rob Sandeski, Manager of the Human Body Donation Program

Cadaver staff ensure that the entire process of body procurement, preparation, and use runs smoothly. When a person who is considering becoming a donor first reaches out to the program, they are greeted by a program administrator who provides them with more information, and the program manager will communicate with them and their family to discuss consent and manage expectations around what will happen when the donor dies. When the donor dies, staff must communicate with the Inspector of Anatomy and decide whether the donor is accepted into the program (which is often a matter of storage capability); if so, they organize transportation by an appropriate service. They also oversee the safe storage of bodies and meticulous maintenance of inventory records.

Bodies are also embalmed and prepared to service the needs of the educational program. While cadavers are presented to learners and teachers when they are cleaned, prepared, and draped for a procedure, cadavers arrive to cadaver staff in whatever form they died in. It is up to them to make the cadavers more visually "presentable" and as "lifelike" as possible. This contributes to students' experiences not only because it improves the physical fidelity of the cadaver, but also because it minimizes the discomfort learners will feel when encountering a dead body.

Staff work closely with teachers, constantly identifying ways to improve their educational impact – for instance, by preparing the body to visualize or manipulate the cadaver in specific ways. For example, cadavers must be presented in specific ways to help students visualize whether or not they have correctly intubated a cadaver. Preparing this presentation requires staff to cut open a window in the chest wall that displays the lungs inflating and deflating with bag-mask ventilation.

And while cadaver-based education is deeply concerned about the use and presentation of the body, staff must also attend to issues of safety for staff, students, and teachers. As the chemicals involved in embalming and cadaver preparation are highly flammable, a fire marshal is involved to ensure proper precautions are in place. Because cadavers carry the risk of infectious disease, they need to be pre-screened before their acceptance in the program, and appropriate protective clothing needs to be worn while working with cadavers.

There is an immense level of pride and attention that goes into creating these teaching materials for the students and ensuring that they have the best experience possible. And there is also a personal aspect of this work that is foundationally important. For Rob, another core aspect of his work is the relationship he has with the families of donors:

I was a funeral director before coming to Dalhousie, and in that work, I learned how to interact with families who were grieving the death of a loved one. As the person who was being trusted with their loved one, there is no other responsibility that I care more about.

Before a donor dies, there are many phone calls and a lot of coordinating that needs to be done. Some don't agree with their loved one's wish to donate, which can make things complicated. Other times, the family has questions about how exactly the body will be used and how helpful it will be for students. And then, when the donor dies, we talk to the grieving families again and follow them for a long time afterwards. Inevitably, you end up going from strangers, one phone call, and a few questions ... to now being connected in a very intimate way. It doesn't take long for those roles to change from somebody just off the street to someone you know so much about.

I also help organize the memorial service every year in June, which is a way to both honour the donors and reflect on all we have done during the year. The committal service happens at noon, which is when the ashes or the urns of the donors are all set out with plaques on top. Families will place little mementoes or flowers with the urn. They'll tell us stories. Funny stories, sad stories. People crying, others just happy to share that experience with everybody in that circle. And then, later, we'll reconvene at the church for the memorial service.

There will be a number of people speaking, including the clergy, the head of our department, myself, and a number of students. The names of all the donors will be read out loud. And I think ... when the families are sitting there in a church with 500 other people that made that same choice they did, it's often comforting to them. Knowing that they weren't isolated in those decisions and experiences.

Cadaver work is not neutral. Working with grieving families, organizing a memorial service, supporting students who may be encountering death for the first time, and working with dead bodies on a daily basis requires a tremendous amount of emotional labour. Hence, whether it is through the bureaucratic work of accepting cadavers, the technical work of preparing them, or the emotional work of organizing a memorial service and supporting the people involved in cadaver-based pedagogy, the invisible work of cadaver staff is something that demands to be recognized.

Death and the Underground

When we went down to the basement in Baltimore, there was this man there who was the keeper of the cadavers. In a very blunt way, he said "Down the hall on the right." As we're walking down this long hallway, you'd see photographs of American military personnel, medical personnel training with these cadavers that have been around since probably the late '80s and maybe before. The room where the cadavers were held was full of stretchers and dripping pipes. It was sort of something out of a movie ... a spooky movie.

– George Kovacs

In our ethnographic work with the HBD program and CBS,[26] our observations spoke of the eeriness of the spaces we entered. Cadaver work often happened in basements or tucked-away offices, out of sight from the broader medical school community. Physically and figuratively, much of cadaver work seemed to happen underground.

If we see our practices as historically situated, it makes sense that cadaver work would largely occur behind the scenes. The idea of working with dead bodies has often been a source of deep discomfort within societies. Today, with more and more HBD programs only accepting bodies that were generously given to them by willing participants, body donation is seen as the ultimate act of altruism and kindness.[27] Around the world, memorial ceremonies are held to honour the donors and the generous gift they offered,[22,28,29] and students are invited to express gratitude for the sacrifice the donors and their families made for the sake of their education.

However, the work of those involved in body donation still occurs behind the scenes – perhaps, in part, because of a larger reluctance within society to talk about death.[30] This might be especially salient within a field that aims to resist death and dying.[31] Encountering a cadaver risks being a "mortality cue"[32] for individuals, which some fear may contribute to death anxiety.[33] Perhaps for this reason, stigma still exists around those who work with the dead.[33]

Death, however, is an inevitable part of medicine. And, importantly, those involved in HBD accomplish skilful, compassionate, and noble work that allows not only for a unique educational experience for learners, but for the profound recognition of the gift given by donors. The tasks in which these workers are engaged – whether bureaucratic, technical, educational, or emotional – always involves celebrating the humanity of the cadaver and expressing respect for the person. This work, we argue, deserves to be seen.

Concluding Thoughts

The people involved in human body donation and cadaver-based pedagogy hold essential roles. They are those who develop and implement innovations, who manage the intake and use of cadavers, who talk to families and students about death and dying, and who organize ceremonies to celebrate the lives of the donors. Perhaps due to long-standing stigma around cadaveric dissection and a larger societal discomfort around death, their contributions have largely remained unseen and unacknowledged. However, the dedication and expertise of those who work within this program are foundational to medical education.

Additional Reading

Kovacs, G., Levitan, R., and Sandeski, R. 2018. Clinical cadavers as a simulation resource for procedural learning. *AEM Education and Training*, 2(3), 239–247. https://doi.org/10.1002/aet2.10103

MacLeod, A., Cameron, P., Luong, V., Kovacs, G., Patrick, L., Fredeen, M., Kits, O., and Tummons, J. 2022. Negotiating humanity: an ethnography of cadaver-based simulation. *Advances in Health Sciences Education*, 28, 181–203. Advance online publication. https://doi.org/10.1007/s10459-022-10152-4

MacLeod, A., Luong, V., Cameron, P., Kovacs, G., Fredeen, M., Patrick, L., Kits, O., and Tummons, J. 2022. The lifecycle of a clinical cadaver: Aa practice-based ethnography. *Teaching and Learning in Medicine*,

34(5), 556–72. Advance online publication. https://doi.org/10.1080/10401334.2022.2092111

Prentice, R. 2013. *Bodies in Formation: An Ethnography of Anatomy and Surgery Education. Education.* Duke University Press.

Dyer, G.S.M., and Thorndike, M.E.L. 2000. Quidne mortui vivos docent? The evolving purpose of human dissection in medical education. *Academic Medicine,* 75(10), 969–979. https://doi.org/10.1097/00001888-200010000-00008

Thompson, W. 1991. Handling the stigma of handling the dead: Morticians and funeral directors. *Deviant Behavior,* 12(43), 403–429. https://doi.org/10.1080/01639625.1991.9967888

References

1. Dyer, G.S.M., and Thorndike, M.E.L. 2000. Quidne mortui vivos docent? The evolving purpose of human dissection in medical education. *Academic Medicine,* 75(10), 969–79. https://doi.org/10.1097/00001888-200010000-00008

2. Elizondo-Omaña, R.E., Guzmán-López, S., and de Los Angeles García-Rodríguez, M. 2005. Dissection as a teaching tool: past, present, and future. *The Anatomical Record,* 285B(1), 11–15. https://doi.org/10.1002/ar.b.20070

3. Brenna, C.T.A. 2021. Post-mortem pedagogy: a brief history of the practice of anatomical dissection. *Rambam Maimonides Medical Journal,* 12(1), 1–5. https://doi.org/10.5041/RMMJ.10423

4. Estai, M., and Bunt, S. 2016. Best teaching practices in anatomy education: a critical review. *Annals of Anatomy,* 208, 151–7. https://doi.org/10.1016/j.aanat.2016.02.010

5. Prentice, R. 2013. *Bodies in Formation: An Ethnography of Anatomy and Surgery Education.* Duke University Press.

6. Kovacs, G., Levitan, R., and Sandeski, R. 2018. Clinical cadavers as a simulation resource for procedural learning. *AEM Education and Training,* 2(3) 239–47. https://doi.org/10.1002/aet2.10103

7. Song, Y.K., and Jo, D.H. 2021. Current and potential use of fresh frozen cadaver in surgical training and anatomical education. *Anatomical Sciences Education,* 15(5), 957–69. https://doi.org/10.1002/ase.2138

8. Thiel, W. 1992. *Die Konservierung ganzer Leichen in natürlichen Farben* [The preservation of the whole corpse with natural color]. *Annals of Anatomy,* 174, 185–95. https://doi.org/10.1016/s0940-9602(11)80346-8

9. Homma, H., Oda, J., Sano, H., Kawai, K., Koizumi, N., Uramoto, H., Sato, N., et al. 2019. Advanced cadaver-based educational seminar for trauma surgery using saturated salt solution-embalmed cadavers. *Acute Medicine & Surgery,* 6(2), 123–30. https://doi.org/10.1002/ams2.390

10. Wannatoop, T., Ratanalekha, R., Wongkornrat, W., Keorochana, K., and Piyaman, P. 2022. Efficacy of a perfused cadaver model for simulated trauma resuscitation in advanced surgical skills training. *BMC Surgery*, 22(1), 1–9. https://doi.org/10.1186/s12893-022-01754-1

11. Rashidian, N., Willaert, W., Giglio, M.C., Scuderi, V., Tozzi, F., Vanlander, A., D'Herde, K., Alseidi, A., and Troisi, R.I. 2019. Laparoscopic liver surgery training course on Thiel-embalmed human cadavers: program evaluation, trainer's long-term feedback and steps forward. *World Journal of Surgery*, 43(11), 2902–8. https://doi.org/10.1007/s00268-019-05103-x

12. Flack, N.A.M.S., and Nicholson, H.D. 2018. What do medical students learn from dissection? *Anatomical Sciences Education*, 11(4), 325–35. https://doi.org/10.1002/ase.1758

13. Jeyakumar, A., Dissanayake, B., and Dissabandara, L. 2019. Dissection in the modern medical curriculum: an exploration into student perception and adaptions for the future. *Anatomical Sciences Education*, 15, 1–15. https://doi.org/10.1002/ase.1905

14. MacLeod, A., Luong, V., Cameron, P., Kovacs, G., Fredeen, M., Patrick, L., Kits, O., and Tummons, J. 2022. The lifecycle of a clinical cadaver: a practice-based ethnography. *Teaching and Learning in Medicine*, 34(5), 556–72. https://doi.org/10.1080/10401334.2022.2092111

15. Yang, J.H., Kim, Y.M., Chung, H.S., Cho, J., Lee, H.M., Kang, G.H., Kim, E.C., Lim, T., and Cho, Y.S. 2010. Comparison of four manikins and fresh frozen cadaver models for direct laryngoscopic orotracheal intubation training. *Emergency Medicine Journal*, 27, 13–16. https://doi.org/10.1136/emj.2008.066456

16. Cullinane, D.P., and Barry, D.S. 2022. Breaking the norm: anatomical variation and its key role in medical education. *Anatomical Sciences Education*, 15(4), 803–5. https://doi.org/10.1002/ase.2141

17. MacLeod, A., Luong, V., Cameron, P., Kovacs, G., Patrick, L., Tummons, J., and Kits, O. 2021. When I say ... human. *Medical Education*, 55(9), 993–4. https://doi.org/10.1111/medu.14537

18. Gunderman, R.B., and Wilson, P.K. 2005. Exploring the human interior: the roles of cadaver dissection and radiologic imaging in teaching anatomy. *Academic Medicine*, 80(8), 745–9. https://doi.org/10.1097/00001888-200508000-00008

19. Chytas, D., Piagkou, M., Salmas, M., and Johnson, E.O. 2020. Three-dimensional digital technologies in anatomy education: better than traditional methods, but are they better than cadaveric dissection? *Clinical Anatomy*, 34(8), 1122–3. https://doi.org/10.1002/ca.23591

20. Riederer, B.M. 2016. Body donations today and tomorrow: what is best practice and why? *Clinical Anatomy*, 29(1), 11–18. https://doi.org/10.1002/ca.22641

21. Taranikanti, V. 2020. Is COVID era the beginning of a paradigm shift in anatomy education? *Medicine & Health*, 15(2), 1–2. https://doi.org/10.17576/mh.2020.1502.01

22. Chang, H.J., Kim, H.J., Rhyu, I.J., Lee, Y.M., and Uhm, C.S. 2018. Emotional experiences of medical students during cadaver dissection and the role of memorial ceremonies: a qualitative study. *BMC Medical Education*, 18(1), 1–7. https://doi.org/10.1186/s12909-018-1358-0

23. Biasutto, S.N., Molina Vargas, I.E., Weigandt, D.M., Mora, M.V., Vargas, R.A.A., Bertocchi Valle, A.J., et al. 2019. Reactions of first year medical students in the dissection room, with prosected corpses, and the incidence on own body donation. *Revista Argentina de Anatomía Clínica*, 11(1), 18–29. https://doi.org/10.31051/1852.8023.v11.n1.23429

24. Douglas-Jones, R. 2017. "Silent mentors": donation, education, and bodies in Taiwan. *Medicine Anthropology Theory*, 4(4), 69–98. https://doi.org/10.17157/mat.4.4.454

25. Olejaz, M. 2017. When the dead teach: exploring the post-vital life of cadavers in Danish dissection labs. *Medicine Anthropology Theory*, 4(4), 125–49. https://doi.org/10.17157/mat.4.4.310

26. MacLeod, A., Cameron, P., Luong, V., Kovacs, G., Patrick, L., Fredeen, M., Kits, O., and Tummons, J. 2022. Negotiating humanity: an ethnography of cadaver-based simulation. *Advances in Health Sciences Education*, 28, 181–203. https://doi.org/10.1007/s10459-022-10152-4

27. Jones, T.W., Lachman, N., and Pawlina, W. 2014. Honoring our donors: a survey of memorial ceremonies in United States anatomy programs. *Anatomical Sciences Education*, 7(3), 219–23. https://doi.org/10.1002/ase.1413

28. Pawlina, W., Hammer, R.R., Strauss, J.D., Heath, S.G., Zhao. K.D., Sahota, S., Regnier, T.D., Freshwater, D.R., and Feeley, M.A. 2011. The hand that gives the rose. *Mayo Clinic Proceedings*, 86(2), 139–44. https://doi.org/10.4065/mcp.2010.0625

29. Kastenbaum, R. 2012. *Death, Society, and Human Experience*, 11th ed. Routledge.

30. Mohd Slim, M.A. 2013. The superhero mythos: a medical student's experience of death. *Journal of Palliative Medicine*, 16(7), 803–5. https://doi.org/10.1089/jpm.2012.0479

31. Wolf, J.J., McVeigh, J., Vallières, F., Hyland, P., and MacLachlan, M. 2020. Death anxiety, self-worth, and exposure to human donor remains: a longitudinal study of Irish medical students. *Death Studies*, 46(4), 875–84. https://doi.org/10.1080/07481187.2020.1783030

32. Tassell-Matamua, N. 2013. Near-death experiences and the psychology of death. *Omega*, 68(3), 259–77. https://doi.org/10.2190/OM.68.3.e

33. Thompson, W. 1991. Handling the stigma of handling the dead: morticians and funeral directors. *Deviant Behavior*, 12(4), 403–29. https://doi.org/10.1080/01639625.1991.9967888

4 The Invisible Work of Simulated Patients and Medical Actors

RICKI LYNÉE, RALPH ALBERTO-MARMOL,
BETH BARRON, AND JONATHAN AMIEL

Students encounter us – and our bodies – to learn how to assess and examine the patient in front of them. Their nerves come up. So, we, as teachers, must think about the learners and their needs, their future patients and their needs, and ourselves and our needs. We each come with our own lived experience, so sometimes we will take a moment to take a pause and make sure that there is safety for everyone involved and that there is the right environment for safety. We think about trauma-informed care. We're here to teach and to make those moments easier, and it becomes part of the work to help learners be sensitive and cognizant of how the simulated patient feels so they can extend the same kindness to their future patients.

– Ricki Lynée, simulated patient

When we invoke simulation to bring education to life, we think about how a learner needs to weave together knowledge, skill, and values in an interpersonal frame in which she or he has enough safety to take risks and reflect on what works well and what needs additional effort. Centring the learner in this way is critical, and yet sometimes we lose a little sight of all that simulation really entails.

In suspending disbelief, we sometimes forget about the individuals who come together to create the simulation for the benefit of the learner, including the authors of the case, the team involved in debriefings, the teachers who prepare the learner for the simulation, and, of course, the simulated patient. We forget about the actors themselves in part because we try to experience them not as actors but as patients, and in part because our focus as educators tends to be on the physician-learners and their needs. But the actors who populate our simulations bring their lived experience, talent, and commitment to their roles every day. When we tune in to their hidden voices, we learn a great deal about what is *actually* happening in a simulation.

In this chapter, we will take a behind-the-scenes look at the role of the simulated patient. Who are these individuals? What influences their participation in this work? What challenges do they navigate and why do they believe this modality is crucial for the training of our learners? What is the experience of the learner? How do simulated patients work with medical school faculty?

To answer these questions, we assembled an author group of an experienced actor and simulated patient (RL), an early medical student (RAM), a faculty member overseeing simulated patient education (BB), and a faculty member working in faculty development and education scholarship (JA). In addition to these professional identities, the author group is diverse in dimensions of identity including age, gender, race, ethnicity, sexuality, and immigration experience. This is particularly important in our effort to frame simulation as a co-constructed and complex experience that brings together professional work with personal histories and perspectives.

We bring the perspectives of the history of simulated patients and the lived experiences of the actor, the learner, and the faculty educator together to illustrate the complexity of the simulation environment and the multiple identities that create it. Though traditionally we have thought of these environments as controlled and reproducible, there is richness in the multiple subjectivities that interact in each encounter that makes them unique and powerful. These inter-subjective dynamics also create the potential for harm through biased assessment and behaviour; thus, they have to be made visible and vigilantly managed.

Simulated Patients: An Academic Perspective

Simulated patients (SPs), also called programed patients or standardized patients, have become a mainstay in medical education over the past half-century. SPs are actors who have been trained to simulate patients with specific medical conditions and a standardized emotional response, creating a predictable environment for medical students to practise their clinical skills.[1]

The use of SPs in medical education dates to the early 1960s, when the University of Southern California School of Medicine developed a program using simulated patients to teach medical interviewing skills to third-year medical students on their neurology clerkship.[1,2] The first simulated patient was named Patty Duggar and she was trained to demonstrate not only the physical signs of multiple sclerosis (paraplegia, sensory loss, monocular blindness, and even Babinski signs), but also the worry that the patient may have in a clinical encounter.

Initially, programs using SPs were criticized for substituting clinical experiences by proxy for experiences with real patients. However, driven largely by a wish for psychometric validity that was not evident in the oral examination practices of the time, other medical schools began to adopt the concept of using SPs into their curricula.[3] The mindset at the time was that by reducing variation between patients, SP-based programs could also reduce variation in learner exposure and assessment for clinicians-in-training.

As the use of SPs continued to gain momentum, the multi-station SP-based Objective Structured Clinical Examination (OSCE) and the Clinical Performance Examination were developed.[4-6] Licensure and credentialing bodies including the Educational Commission for Foreign Medical Graduates and the National Board of Medical Examiners and professional boards including the American Board of Internal Medicine began to pilot programs to train standardized patients for use in certification.[3,7]

In the past 30 years, SP programs have become a ubiquitous element of simulation-based education for medical students and residents.[8,9] The early hope that SP-based OSCEs would become the gold standard for clinical skills assessment is now a point of some contention. Though the 10-station OSCE using highly trained SPs demonstrated a degree of psychometric validity that is compelling for many, others remind us that there are significant theoretical and practical limitations in the degree to which results can be expected to predict clinical performance in real-life settings.[10]

These limitations are also opportunities to consider the simulated patient role in a different light: embracing the inter-subjective experience between actor and learner to explore the way they influence one another and what they learn from one another in doing this work.

Simulated Patients: An Actor's Perspective

> *As SPs, we love what we do and when we meet a learner who is passionate, who wants to learn from their experience with us and to challenge themselves to grow, all in the service of being a good agent for their patients, it feels so good. The commitment on both ends is so important to make for a successful learning experience. Learners who open themselves up, take risks, and have their aha moments are the ones who get the most from this kind of work. Our work is to help them get there.*
> — Ricki Lynée

I'm an actress, writer, producer, and actor-educator from Queens, New York. My parents are from Barbados, so my four siblings and I are first-generation Americans. I've been acting professionally for over 12 years. In simulation, I think of myself as an actor-educator. I started working as an SP six or seven years ago when I met an actress named Linda Freund performing in a production of *Romeo and Juliet* one summer. I thought that using my skills towards the training of doctors and other health professionals was a phenomenal opportunity, so a few weeks after our introduction, I came to the medical centre and started training for this new role. This work felt so right, like I'd found an additional purpose in making a difference, but it certainly took some time to get used to.

What is different in being an SP compared to my role on stage is thinking deeply about what the learner in front of me needs. The training stressed this different perspective. For us to do this work, we not only get into our roles, but we must think very clearly about what we notice about learners 'communication skills, how we provide feedback, how to be intentional in our use of language so that learners can take in what we should add and get excited about their own growth. We also learn about the physical examination and which findings we can simulate.

When I started doing the work, I initially thought I had to have a word-for-word fidelity to the case. But over time, and with experience, I realized that I was focused on internalizing the character and who they are and responding to the learners in ways that feel authentic to who the patient would be. That means there ends up being a lot of variability in what I do from learner to learner, but the coherence is in the character's identity and concerns, and what underlies how they respond to the learners.

One thing that ends up being very important in helping me prepare for an SP session is the orientation I receive about where the learners are in their training, what has come before, and what we are focusing on in this encounter. We'll often be reminded that the learners are nervous and want to do so well. We see that and think about what they need to be working on at this stage of training, and why. That can be communication skills in general, performing the physical examination, motivational interviewing, shared decision-making, and, sometimes, remediation of a particular skill with which the learner is struggling.

When the session begins, what I have to keep in mind are the particulars of the case, how the patient would respond to different choices the learner might make, specific recollections of how the learner is interacting with me, and examples I could bring up in feedback to illustrate to the learner what they did well and the areas in which they may have struggled. That's a lot to keep in mind at the same time, all while portraying a person in a naturalistic way. It's a lot of fast information processing, but once we're familiar with the particulars of the case, we have bandwidth to focus our attention on the learner. Often after the sessions, when the learners have a moment to relieve themselves of all the nerves built up from the idea of working in a testing environment, they often eagerly await to hear my feedback on the areas where they can improve, even more so than the areas in which I felt they excelled. I've become very passionate about this part of the work. It's where I take hold of a direct opportunity to meet the learners 'needs and educate them on the ways that they can greatly enhance the experience for the patient, methods that they can put into practice with me in the moment and implement going forward.

As I have grown in this work, I've realized that the simulated patient role draws on a very particular method for acting. On the stage, we work to elicit certain responses from the audience and to have them understand a story in a particular way. In the simulation centre, we try to be as naturalistic as possible and tune in to the responses the learner elicits from us. This is particularly hard when we are simulating some of life's most difficult moments. For example, people amid depression and experiencing suicidal thoughts, portraying the family member and proxy for a patient who is at the end of life, or the parent of a child who experienced a medical error. Here we bring together intense anxieties that patients experience with those that often elicit a lot of tension in the learners. In these heavy moments, being able both to portray the moment in a compelling way and to be open to the learners 'reactions can be a real challenge. Dealing with trauma in a kind and helpful way is one of our greatest challenges and yet one of the most important things we do.

The other challenge we should bear in mind on a regular basis is tuning into our own blind spots. We are assessing learners and giving them feedback. And we are all different and have our own lived experience. So being vigilant about our implicit biases, and those of our learners, is an important and challenging part of this work. For example, do some learners communicate differently with me, a Black woman, compared to my white colleagues, or colleagues who are men? Do I relate or assess learners differently depending on their race, gender, or other identities?

This work calls for us to tune in to our identities and, in fact, that variety makes the work so rich. But what we need to ensure is that the feedback we provide is based on what we observe right there in the room rather than in preconceived notions or stereotypes about learners. We talk a lot about this, and I think we manage that responsibility well.

Simulated Patients: A Learner's Perspective

Medical students come from all different walks of life that make each of us unique. Some of us have had experiences that prepared us to have a deeper understanding of physician-patient interactions than others. Working with SPs offers us all a chance to practise our communication and clinical skills and, ultimately, to level the playing field so that students who have had virtually no clinical experiences before medical school can catch up to those who have.

– Ralph Alberto-Marmol, medical student

I am a first-generation college student who immigrated to the United States right before starting elementary school. My family is from the Dominican Republic and, as is true for many immigrants in the US, my upbringing presented many challenges that most of my peers did not have to consider. With my acceptance into a medical school situated in a Dominican American neighbourhood came the reassuring feeling that I would learn how to become a doctor in a community that felt like home. However, as grateful as I am to be able to learn within a community that reflects my heritage, I have always worried about how my upbringing would affect my ability to engage in physician-patient interaction. As someone who grew up with limited emphasis on healthcare and who seldom went to the doctor, I felt that I lacked a necessary understanding of what an exchange between a patient and healthcare provider is supposed to look like. I feared that this would later translate to a weakened ability to communicate with the patients that I would soon have to treat.

I was unsure of what working with an SP would entail. We were given simple instructions: treat the SPs as if they were real patients. Immediately, I recognized the value these simulations would have on my medical education. In combination with the lack of familial prioritization of healthcare during my childhood, I also missed out on the opportunity to build my skills in patient interaction during my undergraduate education due to the COVID-19 pandemic. Working with SPs has given me the chance to develop these skills as a medical professional. The SPs not only taught me the importance of adaptability and attentiveness, it also allowed me to understand the patient's perspective of my communication and physical examination skills through the feedback following each interview. What has been really important is that the SPs bring their full selves to the simulations, so thinking about what they are doing and experiencing their ability to step out of role to let us know what they experienced and share their feedback with us has been an incredible learning experience.

The setup of SP interviews and physical examinations contributes to its overall success in simulating patient interactions. There is a real feel of seriousness that a typical patient interaction has, while simultaneously relieving some of the pressure by cultivating an environment in which mistakes are treated as learning opportunities. Moreover, the SPs prioritize an atmosphere that is conducive for learning. Medical students are allowed to ask the preceptor questions throughout the interview, and there is a lot of cognitive processing required to make the SP interview successful. The student is required to engage in intent listening while simultaneously formulating follow-up questions that provide information on a possible diagnosis. The interviews present a space where students can focus on developing their ability to balance these abilities without the added layer of pressure of making mistakes with a real patient. In the physical examinations, we can practise our manoeuvres, explore how we as clinicians touch our patients 'bodies, and how to integrate asking questions, responding to our patients 'questions, and gathering information through physical examinations. These are such new experiences for students, and being able to do this with actors who are trained, patient, and create a safe environment is a real gift.

Working with SPs has motivated me to continue building my skills beyond the classroom. After developing a feel for what the patient interviews typically look like, I was able to emulate these interactions on my own time with some of my peers through role plays. The additional practice allowed me to develop a new level of comfort as a healthcare professional in training, while providing me with the confidence to understand key questions to ask each patient and how to make a patient feel more comfortable in a clinical setting.

In working with SPs, I have been able to hone my interactional skills over just a few months. I can honestly say that I have a deeper understanding of how to engage in patient interactions so that both the patient, and myself as an interviewer, can get the most out of the experience. The interviews have allowed me to determine which areas of patient care I excel at and refine areas that need strengthening. All in all, the SP interviews have been a vital part of my education as a medical student, and I know that the skills I have developed by engaging in these interviews will be skills that I will carry throughout my medical career.

Simulated Patients: An Educator's Perspective

I came into working with SPs as a skeptic. I wasn't sure what these staged experiences could really offer for medical education. But as I got into the work, I saw

how valuable a learning experience this could be and quickly grew incredibly impressed by the work the actors do and how well they bring the patient's voice into the scenarios. The work is incredibly hard. I've tried to be the SP before, and even though I know the symptoms and signs I need to convey without thinking about them twice, the cognitive load of doing that while taking in what the learners are doing, responding to learner behaviours, and then being able to provide feedback in a compassionate and helpful way is incredibly humbling.
– Beth Barron, professor and simulated patient educator

Psychological safety is paramount for the learners, allowing them to trust that they can really lean into this experience, learn from it and know that nothing bad will happen to either them or the patient. While the learners are most focused on the actual experience – i.e., the interviewing and examining of the standardized patient – the most powerful moments of learning, from my perspective, occur during the debriefing of the experience afterwards. While I'm watching the videos with students, they'll notice a moment that concerns them and want to delve deeper into it to brainstorm a different approach. Perhaps it will be a missed opportunity to provide empathy or a response from the patient that was left unexplored.

So many of my conversations with students are about cognitive load. When you're watching a doctor and patient in the room, the conversation appears simple, and you can easily see when there is a disruption in connectedness and empathy. But when you pull back the curtain and start thinking about how much information a doctor needs to think through, how they are prioritizing differentials, how they're responding to patient cues, and how they adapt, you begin to recognize the complexity of the encounter and not only develop an appreciation for the enormity of the task but also humility about what you can expect to accomplish. Much of what I want to help the students learn comes down to being present in the room and listening with as much skill as possible.

The SPs deserve a tremendous amount of respect, collegiality, and recognition that they are core members of the team. I think it's clear that their primary goal is to provide a safe space for learners to practise, but there have been many other benefits to my work with the SPs. The biggest surprise has been how much we can be partners in the cases and case-writing. The actors will identify elements of a case that don't seem realistic, things that someone of a particular age or background wouldn't say, or what points might need more pushback. They help make the cases so much more authentic, and they have taught me to make the cases simpler so that the focus could be on teaching and learning. That is different from real life, when patients may have a much richer and more complex life. Here we can adapt the scenario to focus on specific learning objectives and remove any unnecessary distractions.

The SPs also need to know a lot about who the learners are at this point in their training. They need to know what learners have practised so far, what they've seen before, and what they haven't. They need to understand what my intentions are, what are the stakes, and what ultimately needs to come out of the encounter. All of this helps them to prepare for the expected skill level and to know when they should help the learners and when they shouldn't. They're able to adjust their portrayals and interactions quite skilfully with this information, creating an appropriately challenging encounter.

I do worry about subjectivity and bias in the SPs. Initially, I wanted to believe there is objectivity in the format. But SPs are human beings just like the rest of us, each bringing their own complexity. There are interplays depending on the age, gender, race, and religion of both the SP and the student. While this is clearly true for real patients as well, the intention of these sessions is to obtain the most valid and accurate measure of a student's skills. I am actively working to understand this interplay – how much of an effect does the bias play and where is it most active? How does it affect both portrayal and assessment? Is it most active in highly subjective areas like communication skills and less present in more objective areas (e.g., whether they performed a specific exam manoeuvre)? I try to minimize this bias by watching and regrading videos where scores are unexpectedly low, but I am aware I bring my own biases to this as well. In the end I still think it's an important learning tool, and as with any assessment you need triangulation of data with other sources to try to decrease the effects of any one assessment modality.

There are a lot of opportunities ahead for us, too. Artificial intelligence (AI) is helping us decode narrative assessments in a more efficient and organized way that allows for much richer data to emerge from simulations. And virtual patients are becoming much more realistic and able to generate facial expressions, emotions, and responses in almost real time. I'm really interested in seeing how this evolves but also recognize it takes another step back from the reality of the situation. If the goal of these interactions is to ensure a completely unbiased patient presentation to the learner, then AI can surely support that goal. But SPs do a lot more than just offer a presentation of a patient. They are collaborators in developing the case. They are educators offering feedback to learners. They are critically thinking actors who respond to the learner in appropriate ways, tailored to the learner's unique skill sets. They are making important contributions to medical education. AI will challenge us to think deeply about the role of SPs in medical education. Currently, AI may be a good tool for early or struggling learners to give them more opportunities for practice, but I'm sure more is to come in this area. We need to be ready to harness all of AI's potential while also protecting and maintaining the unique contributions that only SPs can offer.

Concluding Thoughts

In these perspectives, we have shared the perspectives of history and of three individuals who co-create the simulated learning environment. This medical stage brings together the work of the actor, the faculty, and the learner to co-create an educational experience that does not simulate real life but goes further than that. It provides a vital playground for practice, for assessment *for* learning, and for reflection. From an inter-subjective perspective, we can see that each co-creator of this space plays a vital role in shaping its value and the possibility it affords the learner in becoming more skilled and more reflective. As we add critical and constructivist perspectives to the initially positivist framing of a simulation, we learn how much more complex and nuanced the space becomes and how thoughtful and humble we ought to be in its use. This will be particularly important as we deploy newer technologies.

Additional Reading

Abe, K., Roter, D., Erby, L.H., and Ban, N. 2011. A nationwide survey of standardized patients: who they are, what they do, and how they experience their work. *Patient Education and Counseling*, 84(2), 261–4. https://doi.org/10.1016/j.pec.2010.07.017. PMID: 20719464.

Lauckner, H., Doucet, S., and Wells, S. 2012. Patients as educators: the challenges and benefits of sharing experiences with students. *Medical Education*, 46(10), 992–1000. https://doi.org/10.1111/j.1365-2923.2012.04356.x. PMID: 22989133.

Plaksin, J., Nicholson, J., Kundrod, S., Zabar, S., Kalet, A., and Altshuler, L. 2016. The benefits and risks of being a standardized patient: a narrative review of the literature. *Patient*, 9(1), 15–25. https://doi.org/10.1007/s40271-015-0127-y. PMID: 26002043.

References

1. Barrows, H.S., and Abrahamson, S. 1964. The programmed patient: a technique for appraising student performance in clinical neurology. *Journal of Medical Education*, 39, 802–5. PMID: 14180699. https://pubmed.ncbi.nlm.nih.gov/14180699/

2. Barrows, H.S. 1993. An overview of the uses of standardized patients for teaching and evaluating clinical skills. *Academic Medicine*, 68(6), 443–51. https://doi.org/10.1097/00001888-199306000-00002

3. Wallace, P. 1997. Following the threads of an innovation: the history of standardized patients in medical education. *Caduceus*, 13(2), 5–28. PMID: 9509634. https://pubmed.ncbi.nlm.nih.gov/9509634/

4. Harden, R.M., Stevenson, M., Downie, W.W., and Wilson, G.M. 1975. Assessment of clinical competence using objective structured examination. *British Medical Journal*, 1(5955), 447–51. https://doi.org/10.1136/bmj.1.5955.447

5. Barrows, H.S., Williams, R.G., and Moy, H.M. 1987. A comprehensive performance-based assessment of fourth-year students' clinical skills. *Journal of Medical Education*, 62:805–9. https://doi.org/10.1097/00001888-198710000-00003

6. Adamo, G. 2003. Simulated and standardized patients in OSCEs: achievements and challenges 1992–2003. *Medical Teacher*, 25(3), 262–70. https://doi.org/10.1080/0142159031000100300

7. Stillman, P.L., Swanson, D.B., Smee, S., Stillman, A.E., Ebert, T.H., Emmel, V.S., Caslowitz, J., et al. 1986. Assessing clinical skills of residents with standardized patients. *Annals of Internal Medicine*, 105(5), 762–71. https://doi.org/10.7326/0003-4819-105-5-762

8. Colliver, J.A., and Swartz, M.H. 1997. Assessing clinical performance with standardized patients. *JAMA*, 278, 790–1. https://doi.org/10.1001/jama.278.9.790

9. Howley, L.D. 2004. Performance assessment in medical education: where we've been and where we're going. *Evaluation & the Health Professions*, 27(3), 285–303. https://doi.org/10.1177/0163278704267044

10. Hodges, B.A. 2003. Validity and the OSCE. *Medical Teacher*, 25(3), 250–4. https://doi.org/10.1080/01421590310001002836

5 The Invisible Work of Test Administration

ANNA RYAN, KIMBERLEY HOKIN, AND TERRY JUDD

I received an email from a student. They were really anxious about the process and they'd sent me all these questions. "What happens if this happens? What if I do this?" and so on. So I replied, "Do you want to have a chat? Let's have a Zoom and we can chat about the process and the 'what-ifs'." And we just ended up having this great chat, and I was able to dispel some myths and some rumours and say, "You know we're human. We understand that you're human. We understand that it's a stressful time, but there are no trick questions or processes. We're not trying to trip you up. We want you to succeed – we're here for you."

– Kimberley Hokin, former assessment project officer

Assessment in medical education plays a critical role in assuring accrediting organizations, government agencies, and members of the public that our medical students and trainee doctors are work-ready and primed for a lengthy career providing high-quality patient care. While there is clear recognition of the necessity of effective and integrative assessment of medical students' knowledge and skills, and a general consensus on what good assessment looks like, the people involved and processes underpinning assessment in medical education are much less widely acknowledged or appreciated. Some of the key roles of people who operate behind the scenes of medical school exams include:

- Assessment designers
- Item writers
- Quality assurance reviewers
- Exam administrators
- Exam invigilators
- Technical support staff (in the case of online/computer-based assessments)

- Simulated patients and examiners (in the case of OSCEs and related clinical assessments)
- Markers (in the case of written assessments)
- Standard-setting panels
- Data analysts and statisticians
- Feedback developers and providers.

The purpose of this chapter is to highlight some of these people, particularly in the context of modern assessment practice, and reveal how essential their work is for high-quality medical education.

As an author team, we have significant experience in the assessment practices of medical schools, particularly those in Australia. We are all based at the Melbourne Medical School at the University of Melbourne and work intensively in the school's assessment processes. Anna Ryan's interest in assessment began when, as a medical student and then a junior doctor, she felt she was constantly being assessed but that only a fraction of that potentially useful information was being returned to her in a way she could use to improve. This sparked a PhD focused on the impact of progress testing with different types of automated feedback, followed by a program of postdoctoral research focused on assessment for learning, and finally pursuit of a full-time academic medical career. She currently serves as Head of the Department of Medical Education. A trained botanist, Terry Judd has been working and innovating with educational technologies for more than 25 years. Terry's interest and deep involvement in assessment was both sparked and fostered through a very productive and enjoyable working relationship with Anna over the last 10 or so years. Kimberley Hokin first discovered the world of medical assessment while coordinating clinical tutorials and OSCEs for medical students. Since then, Kim has been involved in the implementation of electronic exam delivery in lab, bring your own device, and remote settings. She is passionate about exam integrity, student experience, and ultimately patient safety. As a team, our collective experiences in medical school assessment practices are the foundation of this chapter. The stories of Kim and Terry's work life are the cornerstones of our desire to make visible the work involved behind assessments – work that is often deemed most successful when it goes unnoticed.

An Overview of Assessment in Medical Schools

To understand the work carried out by the many people involved in assessment in medical schools, it is important to consider the history of that assessment work and the many forms of assessment that are now commonplace in medical education. George Miller[1] famously highlighted the complexity of assessment in medical education, claiming that no single assessment tool could "provide all the data required for judgment of anything so complex as the delivery of professional services by a successful physician." This remains true, despite fundamental changes in the design and delivery of medical curricula during the intervening 30 years. Irrespective of the educational models and principles these curricula embody, all rely on the delivery of a combination of assessments focused on knowledge and its application (such as multiple-choice and short-answer question assessments), clinical reasoning and skill (such as the Objective Structured Clinical Examination or OSCE) and engagement in actual clinical practice (such as workplace-based assessments).

Alongside the recognition of the need for multiple assessment formats and modalities has come an increasing recognition that individual assessments should be meaningful and, ideally, authentic to the practice of medicine. They should also be reproducible, feasible, have clear and consistent expectations for learners, be acceptable to invested parties, and make a positive contribution to future learning.[2]

The focus on reproducibility led to the increasing popularity of standardized clinical assessments that sample across a number of cases. The OSCE[3] sees students moving through a series of short "stations," each designed to assess a particular subset of clinical skills. While this sampling approach does improve the reliability of clinical assessment,[4] it involves complex logistics, especially when large student cohorts are involved.[5,6]

A focus on learning, and the growth of the pedagogical and evidence base underpinning feedback practices, has put pressure on traditional paper-based assessment practices.[7] Computer-based assessments allow for more rapid and reliable collection of data and provide far more options for collation and re-presentation of assessment information back to learners. Gone are the days when a learner would (or should) be satisfied by knowing they passed or achieved a certain numeric grade. The expectation now is that each testing moment should be followed with delivery of feedback which is both timely and meaningful for student learning.[2]

More recently, our understanding of effective assessment has broadened beyond a focus on assessment within a single subject or context towards a more integrative or systems approach. While the level of integration may vary, it will typically span multiple knowledge and practice domains and many or all stages of a program or curriculum.

It may even serve to scaffold a learner's entire career journey.[8,9] Such systems or "programmatic" approaches to assessment are most likely to be successful when data from a wide range of assessment types and instances are appropriately and effectively combined. The end goal of this combination should be that staff and students are able to view, interpret, and understand students' progress against clearly defined learning outcomes that are meaningful to students, educators, and accreditation bodies alike.

While gathering data across multiple assessment types and formats, and across multiple years of a curriculum or program, and applying it to inform both learning and progress decisions has very clear value, it is by no means easily achieved. The logistical demands of collecting, collating, and analysing such data and reporting them against a meaningful framework[10] are considerable. Learners also need to be primed so that they are receptive to the findings.[11] Electronic assessment delivery and ePortfolio systems promise solutions to at least some of these issues. However, successfully implementing their affordances in a way that reflects the complexities and nuances of a typical medical curriculum involves many additional challenges.

Mastery of the complex logistics of medical school assessment delivery – as well as the efficient and effective collection, collation, and return of assessment data – have nevertheless become core expectations of assessment within medical education. These two areas are the focus of the remainder of this chapter. The context explored is assessment within an Australian medical school, and the focus is on two roles that are key to the effective and efficient delivery of assessments and the capture, application, and interpretation of assessment data – an assessment project officer and an educational technology academic. In our context, both roles are undertaken by highly skilled staff members who, in the normal course of things, have little direct contact with students as they progress through their medical degree – and therefore remain largely invisible to them and to many staff members.

Test Administration: Delivery of Assessments

The introduction of station-based standardized assessments (such as the OSCE) created a major disruption in medical education. Prior to the development and implementation of OSCEs, clinical assessments had relied on hospital-based encounters involving real patients.[12] The movement of clinical assessments off the wards into controlled environments simultaneously introduced a role (or roles) in coordination of clinical examinations[6] with skills more commonly seen in project management and logistics positions. Titles for these roles vary from site to site and generally reflect the assessment format (e.g., clinical assessment coordinator) or hint at the introduction of a new innovation (e.g., assessment project officer). The people performing these roles in medical school exam circles are affectionately described as "master conductors" or "air traffic controllers." A very similar skill set is currently highly sought after in delivery of computer-based assessments, particularly within those schools transitioning from traditional paper-based to more modern computer-based assessment.

Kimberley Hokin is the master conductor of our medical school's computer-based written exams. She has previously fulfilled a similar role at a specialty college, and prior to that she coordinated clinical exams (OSCEs) at another medical school. Kim is the super-organized person every medical school needs – i.e., someone capable of developing and implementing exam procedures that ensure that students are well supported, that the many academic and professional staff assisting clearly understand and effectively carry out their individual roles, and that exam day goes as smoothly as possible for everyone involved. Kim's passion for this large-scale logistical and management work is clear:

> *For me, and I think probably for anyone who's involved in exam delivery, there's an element of thrill to it. Large-scale exams are a massive undertaking. Everyone has their part to play and it's my job to make sure people know where their role starts and ends. I always say to those involved that it is essential to concentrate on their task alone, because as soon as you move out of your lane to start telling someone else what to do, something inevitably pops up in your own area and you've totally missed it. It's very procedural, but I like that. I like the level of coordination required – ensuring that all the cogs fit and are working together.*
>
> – Kimberley Hokin, assessment project officer

While the combination of high-stakes assessments and the complex logistics required to coordinate students, examiners, and support staff on exam days would be enough to paralyse many, Kim takes immense satisfaction from successfully navigating the practical and administrative challenges involved:

> *When I was responsible for OSCEs at my previous medical school, we were running them in an historic building – a 1900s warehouse. It had multiple internal levels, each of which had been converted into clinical spaces, tutorial rooms, and offices. We ran large multi-station OSCEs where students were all going up and down stairs, down there and around here as they moved between their stations.*

You needed to keep close track of them the whole way. And even before you get to that point there's the setting up of all the rooms, the beds, the equipment, making sure all the examiners and simulated patients are in the right place and know what they are supposed to be doing. The logistics were crazy, but I loved it.

– Kimberley Hokin

Some of Kim's largest challenges, and greatest achievements, have arisen from the transition of her current and previous workplaces from paper to computer-based assessments. While on the face of it this might appear to reduce some or much of the logistical and administrative complexity around exam delivery – particularly when it comes to post-exam data capture and processing – in reality it introduces a whole new set of challenges:

When I was working for the specialist medical college, we were running our written exams in dedicated testing centres. Some exams were on paper, but increasingly they were being delivered electronically in large computer labs. There were a number of different specialties covered within the college and each had its own "special" requirements in how they wanted assessments delivered. Some were delivered via paper, some were delivered electronically, and some a mix of both. Often exams required ultra specific formatting. For example, [X specialty] loved including images in their items – pretty much every item revolved around an image. And whether the exam is delivered on paper or electronically, you need to make sure that image looks exactly the same for everyone – the right resolution, the right colour, the right contrast, and so on. The attention to detail required to get that all right when the stakes are so high is incredible.

– Kimberley Hokin

And the challenges are different in relation to each user. With examiners and markers, for example, establishing and maintaining ongoing relationships strong enough to weather fundamental process change is critical.[13] Kim has a deep appreciation for the need to nurture those relationships:

Relationship and trust building was just so important in supporting the college to transition from paper to electronic assessments. There were some initial hiccups with the transition, so it meant there was some resistance to change. From the markers, for example. They're typically busy consultants. They are giving up their precious time to help out. They are used to marking on paper and don't have the time or inclination to familiarize themselves with a new process. For them it's all about the validity and integrity of the exam process and, despite its inherent inefficiencies, they had confidence in the old paper-based processes. Despite this, by building relationships with them and transitioning gradually we were able to successfully change many of our exams from paper to electronic delivery. And this was pre-COVID, so I can confidently claim that we qualified as early-ish adopters of electronic exam delivery and marking.

In retrospect, Kim's initial experience of supporting examiners through the transition from paper to electronic marking at the surgical college was the ideal preparation for the massive changes required in her current role. Melbourne was subjected to some of the longest and most stringent lockdowns worldwide during the first two years of the COVID-19 pandemic,[14] and Kim was at the centre of our rapid pivot to remotely delivered online exams:

The change happened so quickly. I mean COVID hit and we had exams to deliver, and the only way to do that reasonably securely was to go to remote "bring your own device" (BYOD) exams. We'd planned a slow, measured transition to BYOD exams, but this was like everything, everywhere, all at once. And having to go remote, which certainly wasn't part of our original plan, meant having to deal with the whole issue of video invigilation and potential academic integrity breaches. It was really tricky, but in the end that aspect was one of the most interesting parts of the job to me.

While most aspects of Kim's work behind the scenes delivering exams continued to remain largely invisible to students, an unexpected consequence of our rapid pivot to BYOD and remote delivery was that a few aspects of her role – in particular those focused around technology adoption and support – became much more visible to a small subset of students, most notably those students with technical or computer-related queries or issues flagged as part of our academic integrity processes.[15] Kim's handling of these situations highlights, again, the communication savvy that is needed in this kind of work:

In the case of students who had failed to complete an adequate pre-exam environment scan, I'd often show them a screenshot of something they were doing during the exam, like obviously looking away from the screen. At that point most of them would get it – why they had been flagged and what they needed to do – or not do – next time around. Even some of those that start off quite affronted end up getting why they're being contacted and why the process they've unfortunately been caught up in is necessary – to ensure that the exam they are doing has integrity and that the conditions are fair and equal for everyone. That sense of fairness is very important to students.

While Kim enjoyed the change to clarify procedural issues directly with small number of students, her role's low overall visibility does create some challenges. In particular, it carries with it a risk of underestimation of complexity of the task and therefore lack of recognition and support for those involved. On the other hand, as Kim explains, invisibility to students can almost be seen as a marker of success in these kinds of roles:

I think that the visibility or understanding of what my role entails to those who allocate budgets to the running of exams is probably a bit outdated, particularly now that we have transitioned to BYOD delivery. Everyone has experience of exams and has witnessed what goes on around them in an exam venue and probably thinks they have a reasonable idea of who and what is required to run them. Understanding that you need X number of invigilators for Y number of students is one thing, but appreciating the complexity of the processes, and the careful and considered engagement with students – that's another level.

Students, on the other hand – ideally, they shouldn't even be aware of you and what you do. Someone provides them with their exam instructions and there are invigilators keeping an eye on them, but that's about it. From my perspective a boring exam is a good exam.

Test Administration: Making Sense and Use of the Data

Over recent years the development of technological advances impacting on education has increased exponentially,[16] and the area of medical education assessment is no exception.[17,18] Technology is recognized to have an impact across many aspects of assessment, including authenticity, student engagement, design, delivery, tracking of learner achievement, and support of longitudinal and continuous assessment.[18] It requires people with rich expertise to develop and support this work. At some sites this work is done by programmers, learning designers, or experts in educational technology.

Terry Judd is our lead for technology-enhanced assessment. He is an academic with a non-medical background who specializes in learning technologies and their application. Over recent years he has focused primarily on routinely providing students with meaningful post-exam feedback in combination with comprehensive and effective individualized assessment dashboards. Terry's description of this work highlights how the work he does can be used to support our students develop a mastery approach to learning:

Something we've been doing for quite a few years now is to employ and apply learning analytics to produce individualized and detailed feedback reports to students after all of our exams. We are able to achieve this because our written and clinical assessment items are extensively tagged or mapped to their relevant knowledge domains and learning outcomes. This allows us to report each student's performance against those domains, and in the process highlight any emerging – or established – strengths and weaknesses. A high degree of consistency of these reports across our various assessment types, in conjunction with the integrated and longitudinal nature of our assessment program, means that students can use these reports to track their progress within and across the years of their course. Beyond that, though, our real expectation is that they will use that information to help to guide and plan their future learning.

– Terry Judd, Lead for Technology-Enhanced Assessment

Terry and Anna Ryan, co-author of this chapter, started working on the development and production of these reports around 10 years ago. From relatively small-scale and experimental beginnings,[19] the project has grown and evolved across multiple testing formats as the school has progressively moved towards a programmatic approach to assessment across all four years of the medical program.[7,20–23] Bringing this change to fruition required not only the expertise offered by Terry and Anna, but also a spirit of collaboration and a shared commitment to the goal:

Having worked extensively with learning analytics, I was keen to help out with Anna's PhD project and could see the potential that automated feedback on test performance offered. Anna and I worked well together, and my involvement just grew over time. The complexity and scope of the project also grew progressively as we added new ways for students to visualize and interpret their performance data and applied our methodologies to more assessment types and formats. Now, all students routinely receive these reports after each of their exams, meaning that we produce batches of around 350 individualized reports about 25 times a year. While much of the process is automated, it still requires a reasonable degree of "manual" handling. For example, we need someone to tag the items, pre-process and format the results data, generate the reports, and upload and publish them to students' assessment dashboards alongside their results.

– Terry Judd

The other significant focus of Terry's work has been the progressive adoption and implementation of a course-wide ePortfolio system. The initial implementation in 2021 involved students in only two of the four years of the medical course, but the system now services all students and handles the submission and management of all their workplace-based assessments and written assignments. In addition, Terry has co-opted – and slightly subverted – the system to serve as the repository and "source of truth" for all students' results, including for their written and clinical exams. These data are aggregated at both the individual student level – to populate the various views on individualized assessment dashboards – and also across each year-level cohort to support our decision making around student progression. This work on the ePortfolio system, as with Kim's work on our BYOD exam delivery system, has been central to us successfully transitioning from paper-based to electronic assessment. As Terry explains, this transition has not been without its difficulties:

> *Implementation of the ePortfolio system has definitely had its challenges. The system is great, and very flexible, but with that flexibility comes complexity so that each staff member has access to the right students and the right information with just the right level of functionality and access. There are so many moving parts and so many discrete jobs that need to be completed to set things up each year and to keep it ticking over. It's definitely more than enough to keep one person occupied, and I've shouldered the brunt of that during our establishment phase over the last couple of years.*
>
> *– Terry Judd*

As is the case with much of Kim's work, Terry's effort and the skills required of him to support our feedback delivery and ePortfolio systems stays hidden from the majority of students and staff:

> *As far as our feedback reports go, I'm fairly confident that students have little or no idea of what data are involved or how these are produced and distributed after each exam. They just know to expect that they will receive them and will certainly let us know if the data and their results aren't received in a timely way. The same goes for our ePortfolio system – and I suppose any learning support system, really – it just needs to do its job, be easy to use and navigate and provide access to all the things that students need to do and see. The only time they really interact with us, the people, rather than it, the system, is when something goes wrong or they need some assistance.*
>
> *The same generally goes for staff users, although some, particularly those who have had to work through the change process in moving from paper-based to electronic assessment delivery and management, will likely have a better idea of the sorts of activities that are likely to be going on behind the scenes. But if we get things right, then that awareness should, along with any initial adoption resistance, fade as their use of the system and the processes we have designed to support it become ingrained over time.*
>
> *– Terry Judd*

It would seem that not only should effective learning systems' interfaces embody and conceal the code and logic that underpins them, they should do their best to shield the user from the operational and administrative processes required to make them operational. That hopefully leads to good outcomes and experiences for end users. But it can have downsides for the staff involved, particularly during the initial stages of a system's implementation, as in Terry's case:

> *It might seem a bit unusual for someone with an ostensibly academic role to be so heavily and intimately involved in a large-scale technology implementation, but not perhaps that unusual if your academic specialty is educational technology. That level of involvement definitely comes at a cost, though. The more involved you are, the harder it is to maintain some of the more recognizably academic aspects of your role. After struggling to maintain any real level of research activity for a number of years, I recently made the difficult and, if I'm honest, not entirely welcome decision to change my long-standing work focus classification from teaching and research to teaching specialist.*
>
> *– Terry Judd*

Terry's decision was largely driven by our shift from paper to computer-based assessments and the amount of work, including often low-level administrative work, that entailed. The type of work involved isn't necessarily the problem – all academics are required to carry substantial administrative loads – it's the volume and constancy of the work and the need for it to be supported appropriately over the long term. Large-scale, ongoing system implementations need to be appropriately resourced, which means having the right people with sufficient capacity doing the relevant jobs. But the transition from the initial phase of development and implementation to "business as usual" can be difficult, particularly the handover of routine tasks which don't yet appear routine to those staff tasked with taking them on. Making those aspects of the implementation that need to be managed by someone else *less* hidden – at least to the people responsible for supporting that transition – is something that we are actively working on.

Concluding Thoughts

The roles highlighted in this chapter are non-traditional medical school academic roles, which have arisen out of recent innovations in assessment. While exams and medical curricula have always gone hand in hand, the introduction of standardized clinical assessments and computer-based examinations has created a need for test administrators with skills in logistics and project management, as well as exceptional attention to detail. More programmatic approaches to assessment necessitate collection of vast amounts of assessment data in electronic format, and the collation and meaningful reporting of these data require significant expertise in information management, feedback provision, and educational technologies more generally.

Student appreciation and peer recognition are both important factors in academic job satisfaction,[24] as are discipline-based recognition and intrinsic motivation.[25] However, both academics featured in this chapter agree that they're largely invisible to many – particularly students. And, while both welcome recent gains in the visibility of their roles associated with the implementation and adoption of new technologies – a rapid BYOD exam delivery conversion in response to the COVID-19 pandemic, and recent adoption of a course-wide assessment reporting system – they also acknowledge that these gains are temporary and will be largely lost as these implementations are bedded down. In fact, both Kim and Terry suggest that the invisibility of their roles, particularly to students, is almost a mark of effectiveness in their job.

Kim and Terry suggest a number of reasons why their jobs might be largely invisible. Both, in the normal course of activity, have very little direct contact with students. Their work, with its heavy administrative and logistic components, is primarily conducted away from health service sites and instead is computer based. They don't have direct face-to-face involvement in teaching medical students, and Terry has highlighted how challenging it can be to maintain research productivity in a role like his. In Australian universities, academic roles are typically focused on teaching, research, and administration, and the "typical" workload division in our context is 40 per cent, 40 per cent, and 20 per cent, respectively.[26] Academic recognition usually arises from some kind of measure in each domain. Research outputs are easy to quantify (e.g., number of publications, success on research grants). Likewise, student experience surveys can demonstrate teaching skill and improvement over time, albeit with some significant limitations.[27] Administrative academic work outcomes are arguably the most challenging of all to measure; however, in Kim's and Terry's positions, administrative work takes up an enormous proportion of their time. This highlights the importance of medical schools having some way of recognizing and rewarding this type of essential work through promotion, awards, and prizes.

While Kim and Terry have clearly described elements of the work itself which brings them satisfaction – speaking to their intrinsic motivation – there's another factor that's evident in their responses, and that's their motivation to contribute to the underlying purpose of medical education:

It's definitely a thrill – to play a key part in training those students who will before too long be doctors. And knowing with confidence that you would happily allow your child be treated by them.

– Kimberley Hokin

Additional Reading

Fuller, R., Goddard, V.C., Nadarajah, V.D., Treasure-Jones, T., Yeates, P., Scott, K., Webb, A., Valter, K., and Pyorala, E. 2022. Technology enhanced assessment: Ottawa consensus statement and recommendations. *Medical Teacher*, 44(8), 836–50. https://doi.org/10.1080/0142159X.2022.2083489

Ryan, A., and Judd, T. 2022. From traditional to programmatic assessment in three (not so) easy steps. *Education Sciences*, 12(7), 487. https://doi.org/10.3390/educsci12070487

Wilkinson, T.J., and Tweed, M.J. 2018. Deconstructing programmatic assessment. *Advances in Medical Education and Practice*, 9, 191–7. https://doi.org/10.2147/AMEP.S144449

References

1. Miller, G.E. 1990. The assessment of clinical skills/competence/performance. *Academic Medicine*, 65(9), S63–7. https://doi.org/10.1097/00001888-199009000-00045

2. Norcini, J., Anderson, B., Bollela, V., Burch, V., Costa, M.J., Duvivier, R., Galbraith, R. et al. 2011. Criteria for good assessment: consensus statement and recommendations from the Ottawa 2010 Conference. *Medical Teacher*, 33(3), 206–14. https://doi.org/10.3109/0142159X.2011.551559

3. Harden, R.M., and Gleeson, F. 1979. Assessment of clinical competence using an objective structured clinical examination (OSCE). *Medical Education*, 13(1), 39–54. https://doi.org/10.1111/j.1365-2923.1979.tb00918.x

4. Newble, D. 2004. Techniques for measuring clinical competence: objective structured clinical examinations. *Medical Education*, 38(2), 199–203. https://doi.org/10.1111/j.1365-2923.2004.01755.x

5. Boursicot, K., and Roberts, T. 2005. How to set up an OSCE. *The Clinical Teacher*, 2(1), 16–20. https://doi.org/10.1111/j.1743-498X.2005.00053.x

6. Khan, K.Z., Gaunt, K., Ramachandran, S., and Pushkar, P. 2013. The objective structured clinical examination (OSCE): AMEE guide no. 81. Part II:

organisation & administration. *Medical Teacher*, 35(9), e1447–63. https://
doi.org/10.3109/0142159X.2013.818635

7. Ryan, A., and Judd, T. 2022. From traditional to programmatic assessment
in three (not so) easy steps. *Education Sciences*, 12(7), 487. https://doi
.org/10.3390/educsci12070487

8. Norcini, J., Anderson, M.B., Bollela, V., Burch, V., Costa, M.J., Duvivier,
R., Hays, R., Palacios Mackay, M.F., Roberts, T., and Swanson, D. 2018.
Consensus framework for good assessment. *Medical Teacher*, 40(11), 1102–9.
https://doi.org/10.1080/0142159X.2018.1500016

9. van der Vleuten, C.P., and Schuwirth, L.W. 2005. Assessing professional
competence: from methods to programmes. *Medical Education*, 39(3),
309–17. https://doi.org/10.1111/j.1365-2929.2005.02094.x

10. Wilkinson, T.J., and Tweed, M.J. 2018. Deconstructing programmatic
assessment. *Advances in Medical Education and Practice*, 9, 191–7. https://
doi.org/10.2147/AMEP.S144449

11. Eva, K.W., and Regehr, G. 2013. Effective feedback for maintenance of
competence: from data delivery to trusting dialogues. *Canadian Medical
Association Journal*, 185(6), 463–4. https://doi.org/10.1503/cmaj.121772

12. Stokes, J. 1979. How to do it: take a clinical examination. *British Medical
Journal*, 1(6156), 98. https://doi.org/10.1136/bmj.1.6156.98

13. Weymes, E. 2002. Relationships not leadership sustain successful organisations. *Journal of Change Management*, 3(4), 319–31. https://doi.org/10
.1080/714023844

14. Campbell, D. 2021. Josh Frydenberg says Melbourne is the world's most
locked down city. Is that correct? ABC News 24, October 24. Available
from: www.abc.net.au/news/2021-10-25/fact-check-is-melbourne-most
-locked-down-city/100560172

15. Ryan, A., Hokin, K., Judd, T., and Elliott, S. 2020. Supporting student academic integrity in remote examination settings. *Medical Education*, 54(11),
1075–6. https://doi.org/10.1111/medu.14319

16. Alexander, B., Ashford-Rowe. K., Barajas-Murphy, N., Dobbin, G., Knott,
J., McCormack, M., Pomerantz, J., Seilhamer, R., and Weber, N. 2019.
EDUCAUSE Horizon Report: 2019 Higher Education Edition [Internet]. EDU-
CAUSE. Available from: https://library.educause.edu/-/media/files
/library/2019/4/2019horizonreport.pdf.

17. Amin, Z., Boulet, J.R., Cook, D.A., Ellaway, R., Fahal, A., Kneebone, R.,
Maley, M., et al. 2011. Technology-enabled assessment of health professions education: consensus statement and recommendations from the
Ottawa 2010 conference. *Medical Teacher*, 33(5), 364–9. https://doi.org/10
.3109/0142159X.2011.565832

18. Fuller, R., Goddard, V.C., Nadarajah, V.D., Treasure-Jones, T., Yeates, P.,
Scott, K., Webb, A., Valter, K., and Pyorala, E. 2022. Technology enhanced

assessment: Ottawa consensus statement and recommendations. *Medical Teacher*, 44(8), 836–50. https://doi.org/10.1080/0142159X.2022.2083489

19. Ryan, A. 2015. Post-test feedback: knowledge acquisition & learning behaviours. Doctoral dissertation. University of Melbourne. Available from https://hdl.handle.net/11343/54979

20. Goss, B.D., Ryan, A.T., Waring, J., Judd, T., Chiavaroli, N.G., O'Brien, R.C., Trumble, S.C., and McColl, G.J. 2017. Beyond selection: the use of situational judgement tests in the teaching and assessment of professionalism. *Academic Medicine*, 92(6), 780–4. https://doi.org/10.1097/ACM.0000000000001591

21. Judd, T., Ryan, A., Flynn, E., and McColl, G. 2017. If at first you don't succeed ... adoption of iPad marking for high-stakes assessments. *Perspectives on Medical Education*, 6, 356–61. https://doi.org/10.1007/s40037-017-0372-y

22. Ryan, A., Judd, T., Swanson, D., Larsen, D.P., Elliott, S., Tzanetos, K., and Kulasegaram, K. 2020. Beyond right or wrong: More effective feedback for formative multiple-choice tests. *Perspectives on Medical Education*, 9(5), 307–13. https://doi.org/10.1007/s40037-020-00606-z

23. Ryan, A., McColl, G.J., O'Brien, R., Chiavaroli, N., Judd, T., Finch, S., and Swanson, D. 2017. Tensions in post-examination feedback: information for learning versus potential for harm. *Medical Education*, 51(9), 963–73. https://doi.org/10.1111/medu.13366

24. Houston, D., Meyer, L.H., and Paewai, S. 2006. Academic staff workloads and job satisfaction: expectations and values in academe. *Journal of Higher Education Policy and Management*, 28(1), 17–30. https://doi.org/10.1080/13600800500283734

25. McInnis, C. 1999. *The Work Roles of Academics in Australian Universities* [Internet]. Canberra: Department of Education, Training and Youth Affairs. Available from: http://hdl.voced.edu.au/10707/269243.

26. Miller, J. 2019. Where does the time go? An academic workload case study at an Australian university. *Journal of Higher Education Policy and Management*, 41(6), 633–45. https://doi.org/10.1080/1360080X.2019.1635328

27. Hessler, M., Pöpping, D.M., Hollstein, H., Ohlenburg, H., Arnemann, P.H., Massoth, C., Seidel, L.M., Zarbock, A., and Wenk, M. 2018. Availability of cookies during an academic course session affects evaluation of teaching. *Medical Education*, 52(10), 1064–72. https://doi.org/10.1111/medu.13627

6 Behind the Scenes: The Hidden Work of Medical School Admissions

SARAH BURM, ANDREA RIDEOUT,
AND CAROLYN DOYLE

Sending an email to somebody to say that there's an offer available, there's a seat available in medical school is one thing. It's super exciting. But as we move into the summer and we get closer to registration day, if a seat opens up, we pick up the phone because of just the timing and we want to get an answer. And if they say no, then we want to quickly go to the next person on the list. And this particular year, it was probably, I don't know, my fourth or fifth year working in the admissions office, and I was allowed to make that call. And I think it was the first call I ever made to somebody. And it was very late in the summer. I think we were a week away from registration day. And I picked up the phone and I called this woman, and I said, "It's Carolyn. I'm calling from Dalhousie Medicine. I'm calling to let you know that a seat has opened up." And she burst into tears, and she said, "I can't even believe you're calling me right now." She was in New Brunswick. She said, "I'm literally walking to my car with my suitcase to drive to Halifax to rewrite the MCAT so that I can get a better score to reapply and now I don't have to go." And just that – the fact that that was what was happening in that moment. And she obviously accepted. She was thrilled. Like just a simple phone call is such a significant moment in time with such impact on someone's life, it's always stuck with me.
– Carolyn Doyle, Admissions Administrative Coordinator

What makes a *good* physician? The answer to this question may seem obvious on the surface: most of us expect our medical provider to possess a strong clinical acumen and offer sound healthcare advice. For others, prior healthcare interactions may have us choosing a physician who exhibits "good bedside manner," takes genuine interest in our well-being, and shares aspects of our social identity.

Of course, the characteristics and behaviours that make a good physician are neither finite nor complete, and there is no simple "right answer." How, then, in a profession where one is expected to demonstrate good judgment, respect, and selflessness, are decisions made about who will ultimately be a *good* physician? More specifically, what is the work of a medical school in determining which applicants are likely to be successful in training, and later as a health professional?

In this chapter, we turn a focused eye to how this largely administrative process unfolds at one medical school. We take readers behind the scenes, yielding insight into how these tough choices are made and who the individuals are who work in these hidden spaces to bring these processes to life. While each of us fulfil distinct academic roles within the medical school where we work, we are united by our strong interest in alleviating the structural and sociocultural barriers impeding certain groups from seeking entry to and finding a sense of belonging throughout medical education. Sarah Burm is a PhD education researcher who studies how individuals and institutions engage with calls to advance equity, diversity, inclusion, and accessibility in medical education. Andrea Rideout is a Family Physician and Assistant Dean of Undergraduate Medical Admissions at Dalhousie University; she brings to this chapter an understanding of the invaluable work of medical school admissions as an academic leader. Carolyn Doyle shares her lived experience working as an admissions administrator for more than 10 years. Together, we provide readers with an unheralded account of the invisible labour and service work behind medical school admissions.

Medical School Admissions: An Academic Perspective

There is no sugar-coating it – applying to medical school is a lengthy, expensive, and complex process. It is also an exceedingly competitive one; the number of prospective students vastly outnumbers the seats available.[1] Yet, year after year, medical schools receive an astounding number of submissions from applicants striving towards the same goal: entrance into the medical profession. It is no surprise, then, that the policies and procedures medical schools use to select applicants regularly undergo considerable scrutiny by accrediting bodies, academic partners, and laypersons alike.

What exactly are medical schools looking for when they appraise applicants' suitability for a career in medicine? Interestingly, many aspects of today's admissions criteria can be traced back to *The Flexner Report*. Among the recommendations was endorsement for higher admission and graduation requirements, with the expectation that learners demonstrate proficiency in the scientific method:

> We have concluded that a two-year college training, in which the sciences are "featured" is the minimum basis upon which modern medicine can

be successfully taught. If the requisite number of physicians cannot at one point or another be procured at that level, a temporary readjustment may be required; but such an expedient is to be regarded as a makeshift that asks of the sick a sacrifice that must not be required of them a moment longer than is necessary.[2] (p. 26)

Reliance on academic selection measures, such as grade point averages and MCAT scores, were traditionally thought to provide a more objective, merit-based evaluation of an applicant's readiness for medical school and eventual success in medicine.[3-5] However, considerable debate exists around whether measures of academic performance should play such a dominant role in medical school selection deliberations. Scholars have critiqued medical school admissions processes for over-relying on high academic accomplishment, expressing concerns that they fail to capture the range of competencies needed for medical practice[6] and favour applicants with higher socioeconomic status while disadvantaging those who may not have the social and cultural advantage to access certain educational or extracurricular opportunities.[7-11]

To address these concerns, medical schools have been recalibrating their admission requirements to align with the principles of holistic review. Simply speaking, holistic review refers to "mission-aligned admissions or selection processes that take into consideration applicant's experiences, attributes, and academic metrics as well as the value an applicant would contribute to learning, practice, and teaching."[12] The move towards holistic criteria means many medical schools are now relying on different data sources and evaluation methods to develop a comprehensive understanding of each applicant, such as completion of a narrative writing exercise (e.g., an autobiographical sketch), a situational judgment test (e.g., CASPer), reference letters, and participation in an interview.[13-15] From this vantage point, medical schools are better positioned to evaluate an applicant as a *whole person*. Similarly, applicants can provide a broader picture of their background and skillset by elaborating on personally significant life experiences, activities, or accomplishments, as well as hardships or extenuating circumstances that may have impacted their education trajectory and decision to pursue a career in medicine.

We know, however, that changes to admission requirements alone are not sufficient for improving diversity and inclusivity in the clinical learning environment. Numerous analyses point to the "hidden curriculum of privilege"[16] (p. 45) and the discursive tensions between academia and the medical profession.[17-20] Recognizing this, medical schools have implemented multiple interventions to optimize equity in admissions outcomes, such as establishing pipeline and pathway programs to support prospective or current students seeking a career in medicine,[21,22] improving and enhancing community engagement throughout undergraduate medical education,[23] and introducing implicit bias and cultural sensitivity training for those involved in admissions decisions.[15]

Now that we have outlined the specific criteria medical schools are looking for when reviewing applications, let us focus on the human actors involved in medical school selection. In these next sections we turn our attention to Andrea and Carolyn's own understanding of the process and inner workings of medical school admissions in Canada.

Medical School Admissions: A Physician's Perspective

So, my role is really to oversee the admissions process and communicate the application requirements each year, as well as making sure that we are following the process in a fair and equitable manner. At the same time, I am also keeping up with the most recent activity in literature around admissions requirements and best practices to bring to the admissions committee so that they can deliberate whether current requirements are still appropriate, or require adjustment based on our social accountability responsibilities. And the truth of the matter is that everyone at some point in their life is going to have an experience with the healthcare system and may be a patient. It is my honest belief that as many people as possible should have an opportunity to be involved in selecting who comes into medical school and who eventually becomes a physician in the healthcare system.
– Andrea Rideout, Assistant Dean, Admissions

For every new student admitted to medical school, there are dozens of people working tirelessly behind the scenes to ensure the admissions process unfolds in a fair and rigorous manner. Specifically at Dalhousie University, the medical school admissions committee is made up of 23 members with representation from three main groups: faculty (clinical and non-clinical), students, and community members. Admissions committee members are approved for a fixed term and in accordance with the defined terms of reference of the committee. With support from the admissions office, committee members review and assess personal statements and the supplemental form components of each applicant's file (e.g., extracurricular involvement, volunteer/paid employment etc.). Files are assigned to multiple reviewers, with committee members assigning a weighted score for each of the above-mentioned application components.

These are then combined with the academic and Multiple Mini Interview (MMI) scores to arrive at a summative application score.

In situations where committee members identify a matter of concern, applications are considered as a group. This is a weighty task. Invisible to the public eye is the increasing workload of processing and screening hundreds of applications and the frequent meetings, often undertaken outside working-day hours, to ensure processes and selection criteria are both equitable and accessible. As Andrea explains, it leaves all those involved wanting to ensure that the composition of a medical school not only includes people that have the knowledge, skills, and attributes necessary for developing into a capable physician, but that also reflects societal needs:

> *Understandably, people have lots of thoughts about admissions and who should be able to come into our program. There seems a perception that there's a very specific checklist to identify exactly who should be coming into the program. And it's not that clear cut. It's not wholly objective and there's a lot of grey areas and just like in medicine, we use the best evidence-based tools that we have at our fingertips at the time and continue to learn and grow based on our learning through each cycle.*
>
> *The tricky thing about admissions is that it is trying to predict the future, and it's because we are not expecting you to be a physician when you come in. That's our job as a medical school, to help you develop into a physician. And at the same time, to do that (to help you become a physician) successfully, I do think you need some evidence of a combination of qualities to thrive and succeed in the program ... No process is perfect and that's why we review it each year. But I do think that what we have is fair and equitable and meets the objective of bringing students that will succeed in the program and eventually become good doctors for our communities.*
>
> *– Andrea Rideout*

The unfortunate reality is many applicants who apply to medical school do not receive an admission offer. This can elicit an emotional response among those who have been unsuccessful as well as loved ones within the applicant's inner circle. For those working in admissions, this can mean withstanding the frustrations of those most impacted. While the reasons for not receiving an offer can be due to lack of evidence of sufficient readiness for medical school, it can also be due to the size of the qualified applicant pool for the limited number of available positions. Given her role in the process, Andrea knows all too well that an applicant who is not selected may still be an applicant with qualifications and capabilities to become a physician:

> *There is a lot of emotion tied to being admitted into medical school. When people hear about someone who didn't get in, it's like "Oh but they have a 4.0 GPA and*

they have a high-scoring MCAT and they did well on their interview; – how could this person not have been accepted?" That doesn't mean they are not a wonderful person. Nor does it mean they are not qualified for medical school. What it means is that there is a large pool of applicants who are qualified and can compete for a medical school spot, and we only have a certain number that we can select. The feedback for unsuccessful applicants is to reflect on the past year, your application process, reflect on the things you think you need to improve. Continue to do the activities that interest you and that you think will help develop skills you can then transfer to medical school. Ultimately, the most core skill I think we're looking for is being a lifelong learner in multiple domains of your life.

– Andrea Rideout

Part of the invisible work Andrea and the admissions office perform includes dispelling persistent myths about the medical school admissions process. Yes, academic capacity is important, but it is just one element of the medical school application. The human element is equally important and can give rich context to an applicant's character, perseverance, and empathy for others.

Medical School Admissions: An Administrative Perspective

I started working at Dalhousie in Admissions in 2009. I was hired as a part-time position to start, and I did two and half days a week in the admissions office ... The amount I have learned since 2009 is substantial. There has been lots of changes to staffing and how the office looks since then. I'm still here and I still love it. I feel like every year I love it more and more ... a lot has to do with the people I work with, for sure.

I don't often think that the work I am doing is contributing to the training of future physicians. However, I do feel that the work I am doing is important to ensure that the proper processes are in place to ensure that we're getting the right students to the Faculty of Medicine ... so it's a piece of the puzzle, a piece of the process on their road to becoming a physician.

– Carolyn Doyle, Admissions Administrative Coordinator

Admissions administrators fulfil an integral role within the medical school. They are often the "eyes and ears" of a medical school, privy to information that is sensitive and confidential in nature as well as forthcoming changes in policy. They work closely with a range of people – from busy senior-level administrators to keen medical school applicants, providing organizational support such as scheduling meetings, preparing and distributing meeting agendas, typing up meeting minutes, inducting new staff and committee members, assigning files to committee members for scoring and review, answering calls and emails from prospective students, and much, much more. In the last few years, technological advancements, COVID-19, and increasing calls to advance equity within the medical workforce have shifted the work of admissions administrators tremendously. For Carolyn and the team she works with, this meant streamlining processes and aiding in the design of new admissions pathways:

So, when I first started, one of the things I laugh about now, it's funny to think about, is when I first started, when we would assess the transcript, and we're talking, you know, 1,000 to 1,500 applications, that many transcripts, we would take a paper transcript and a pencil, and we would go and convert the grades by pencil. And then we would take a calculator and we would do the calculation of the GPA on paper with a pencil and eraser. And now everything's automated. The applicant inputs their grades into an online system. The system calculates their GPA. And then we're just looking at the transcript to verify that what they've entered is correct. So, processing-wise, that's been a huge change since I started. We were still doing paper files prior to 2020. And we were really digging our heels in because that was just what we were comfortable with. We didn't want to change. And then COVID really forced us to change. And now the entire application is essentially paperless. Everything is electronic. And another sort of similar piece of that is back when I started, an application was scanned to a disk, and it was distributed to the admissions committee on a scanned disk. So, if you were an admissions committee member, I would say, "Here's your stack of disks of your applicants that you have to look at their application and score." And they put the disk into their computer or whatever, they'd review it, then they'd return the disk to us. Now it's all, again, automated. And a committee member can log into the system from anywhere. They review an application; they submit their scoring online. Just things like that make me really think, wow, look how far we've come. And then in the last ... really the last two years, the steps that we've taken and the work that's been done to implement priority community pathways. The Indigenous admissions pathway, this is the first year for that. And the Black learner admissions pathway is under development, with a lot of work and collaboration with community, and plans to be in place for the upcoming application cycle. And these pathways were certainly never there when I started. And so, the enhanced self-identification process for those groups, and the work that those subcommittees are doing will be really positive and will have a really good impact on the class composites that come in moving forward.

All the work that goes into processing an application from start to finish relies heavily on our staff, and the relationships we have built with volunteers, committee members, and community partners. Without all these individuals we would not be able to admit the excellent students we do.

– Carolyn Doyle

For applicants in particular, admissions administrators are often their first impression of the medical school. Applicants turn to them when they have questions about the application process. Fortunately for Carolyn, connecting with applicants is another major perk of the job:

I love chatting with applicants. You get to know some of them so well over multiple, multiple emails or phone calls or drop-in visits. And so, getting to know an applicant, and then that applicant being successful, and sharing in that joy of this life-changing news that they're getting is probably one of the most, you know, positive and rewarding pieces of the job that I like. And then once they're in, often those students stay connected with admissions. Like they'll come back, and they'll chat with us, and they'll let us know how things are going. And just watching them go through the program and then seeing them graduate, just getting to know like so many, so many students. And knowing that these could be people that could someday be taking care of myself or my family members is really rewarding, for sure.

– Carolyn Doyle

Delivering bad news can be challenging and there are times when Carolyn's interactions with applicants can be heartbreaking, such as when applicants do not receive the admissions offer that they eagerly await. The sting of rejection can trigger a cascade of difficult emotions for applicants, and supporting applicants through their disappointment is another part of the job for Carolyn and her colleagues:

There are always more qualified applicants than we have available positions. And so, somebody who you know has demonstrated that they have met all the requirements but they are not getting an offer simply because there are not enough seats is a difficult conversation to have. We're often the first point of contact for those applicants to voice their frustrations. And so sometimes we get the brunt of that. And sometimes it's anger, it's frustration. It comes to us first. And so being able to have those conversations. And really, most of the time it's just being able to listen to what they have to say. We usually have a box of tissues in our office on decision letter day. It's a day that's filled with many emotions.

– Carolyn Doyle

Oftentimes, the invisibility of this emotional labour goes unrecognized. It seems that a key component of the work admission administrators like Carolyn do is relationship management. They work tirelessly to build strong connections with the people they engage with on a regular basis, be it the people with whom they work, applicants, or the community at large. Doing so helps the admissions office improve its processes, contributing to a successful outcome for both medical schools and the communities they serve.

Concluding Thoughts

Those involved in admissions arguably perform one of the most important roles within medical education: they are responsible for selecting the medical workforce of tomorrow. This is a job that involves a network of people representing various perspectives, including the broader community. It demands countless hours of preparation and commitment, meticulous review and adherence to policies and procedures, and a strong sense of camaraderie among admissions staff, committee members, community partners, and colleagues. The work of admissions is one where many of its contributors don't mind staying in the shadows; in fact, when things are seemingly "invisible," that usually means the elements of their work are functioning optimally. Ultimately, the accomplishments of those involved in admissions are reflected in the excellence of their student classes and graduates as they grow and develop into peers and colleagues.

Key Reading

Maude, J.M., and Kirby, D. 2022. Holistic admissions in higher education: a systematic literature review. *Journal of Higher Education Theory and Practice*, 22(8), 73–80. https://doi.org/10.33423/jhetp.v22i8.5317

Razack, S., Hodges, B., Steinert, Y., and Maguire, M. 2015. Seeking inclusion in an exclusive process: discourses of medical school student selection. *Medical Education*, 49, 36–47. https://doi.org/10.1111/medu.12547

Reiter, H.I., Lockyer, J.I., Ziola, B.I., Courneya, C.A.I, and Eva, K.I. 2012. Should efforts in favour of medical student diversity be focused during admissions or farther upstream? *Academic Medicine*, 87(4), 443–8. https://doi.org/10.1097/ACM.0b013e318248f7f3

References

1. Lin, K.Y., Anspach, R.R., Crawford, B., Parnami, S., Fuhrel-Forbis, A., and De Vries, R.G. 2014. What must I do to succeed? Narratives from the US

premedical experience. *Social Science & Medicine,* 119, 98–105. https://doi
.org/10.1016/j.socscimed.2014.08.017

2. Flexner, A. 1910. *Medical Education in the United States and Canada: A Report
to the Carnegie Foundation for the Advancement of Teaching* [Internet]. The
Carnegie Foundation for the Advancement of Teaching. Available from:
http://archive.carnegiefoundation.org/publications/pdfs/elibrary
/Carnegie_Flexner_Report.pdf

3. Donnon, T., Paolucci, E.O., and Violato, C. 2007. The predictive validity of
the MCAT for medical school performance and medical board licensing
examinations: a meta-analysis of the published research. *Academic Medicine,* 82(1), 100–6. https://doi.org/10.1097/01.ACM.0000249878.25186.b7

4. Julien, E.R. 2005. Validity of the medical college admission test for pre-
dicting medical school performance. *Academic Medicine,* 80(10), 910–17.
https://doi.org/10.1097/00001888-200510000-00010

5. Kreiter, C.D., and Kreiter, Y. 2007. A validity generalization perspective on
the ability of undergraduate GPA and the medical college admission test
to predict outcomes. Teaching and Learning in Medicine, 19(2), 95–100.
https://doi.org/10.1080/10401330701332094

6. Koenig, J.A., Sireci, S.G., and Wiley, A. 1998. Evaluating the predictive
validity of MCAT scores across diverse applicant groups. *Academic Medicine,* 73(10), 1095–106. https://doi.org/10.1097/00001888-199810000-00021

7. Dhalla, I.A., Kwong, J.C., Streiner, D.L., Baddour, R.E., Waddell, A.E., and
Johnson, I.L. 2002. Characteristics of first-year students in Canadian medical schools. *Canadian Medical Association Journal,* 166(8), 1029–35. PMID:
12002979. https://pubmed.ncbi.nlm.nih.gov/12002979/

8. Lucy, C.R., and Saguil, A. 2020. The consequences of structural racism
on MCAT scores and medical school admissions: the past is prologue.
Academic Medicine, 95(3), 351–6. https://doi.org/10.1097/ACM.0000000
000002939

9. Pitre, T., Thomas, A., Evans, K., Jones, A., Mountjoy, M., and Costa, A.P.
2020. The influence of income on medical school admissions in Canada: a
retrospective cohort study. *BMC Medical Education,* 209, 1–10. https://doi
.org/10.1186/s12909-020-02126-0

10. Talamantes, E., Henderson, M.C., Fancher, T.L., and Mullan, F. 2019. Clos-
ing the gap – making medical school admissions more equitable. *New
England Journal of Medicine,* 380(9), 803–5. https://doi.org/10.1056
/NEJMp1808582

11. Young, M.E., Razack, S., Hanson, M.D., Slade, S., Varpio, L., Dore, K.L.,
and McKnight, D. 2012. Calling for a broader conceptualization of
diversity: surface and deep diversity in four Canadian medical schools.
Academic Medicine, 87(11), 1501–10. https://doi.org/10.1097/ACM
.0b013e31826daf74

12. Association of American Medical Colleges. 2023. Holistic review [Internet]. Association of American Medical Colleges. Available from: www.aamc.org/services/member-capacity-building/holistic-review.

13. Grabowski, C.J. 2018. Impact of holistic review on student interview pool diversity. *Advances in Health Sciences Education*, 23(3), 487–98. https://doi.org/10.1007/s10459-017-9807-9

14. Maude, J.M., and Kirby, D. 2022. Holistic admissions in higher education: a systematic literature review. *Journal of Higher Education Theory and Practice*, 22(8), 73–80. https://doi.org/10.33423/jhetp.v22i8.5317

15. Robinett, K., Kareem, R., Reavis, K., and Quezada, S. 2021. A multi-pronged, antiracist approach to optimize equity in medical school admissions. *Medical Education*, 55(12), 1376–82. https://doi.org/10.1111/medu.14589

16. Razack, S., Hodges, B., Steinert, Y., and Maguire, M. 2015. Seeking inclusion in an exclusive process: discourses of medical school student selection. *Medical Education*, 49, 36–47. https://doi.org/10.1111/medu.12547

17. Alexander, K., Fahey Palma, T., Nicholson, S., and Cleland, J. 2017. "Why not you?" discourses of widening access on UK medical school websites. *Medical Education*, 51(6), 595–611. https://doi.org/10.1111/medu.13264

18. Cleland, J.A., Nicholson, S., Kelly, N., and Moffat, M. 2015. Taking context seriously: explaining widening access policy enactments in UK medical schools. *Medical Education*, 49, 25–35. https://doi.org/10.1111/medu.12502

19. Jones, A.C., Nichols, A.C., McNicholas, C.M., and Stanford, F.C. 2021. Admissions is not enough: the racial achievement gap in medical education. *Academic Medicine*, 96(2), 176–81. https://doi.org/10.1097/ACM.0000000000003837

20. Ellaway, R.H., Malhi, R., Bajaj, S., Walker, I., and Myhre, D. 2018. A critical scoping review of the connections between social missions and medical school admissions: BEME Guide No. 47. *Medical Teacher*, 40(3), 219–26. https://doi.org/10.1080/0142159X.2017.1406662

21. Henderson, R.I., Walker, I., Myhre, D., Ward, R., and Crowshoe, L. 2021. An equity-oriented admissions model for Indigenous student recruitment in an undergraduate medical education program. *Canadian Medical Education Journal*, 12(2), e94–9. https://doi.org/10.36834/cmej.68215

22. Sadler, K., Johnson, M., Brunette, C., Gula, L., Kennard, C., Charland, D., Tithecott, G., et al. 2017. Indigenous student matriculation into medical school: Policy and progress. *International Indigenous Policy Journal*, 8(1), 1–15. https://doi.org/10.18584/iipj.2017.8.1.5

23. Strasser, R., Worley, P., Cristobal, F., Marsh, D.C., Berry, S., Strasser, S., and Ellaway, R. 2015. Putting communities in the driver's seat: the realities of community-engaged medical education. *Academic Medicine*, 90(11), 1466–70. https://doi.org/10.1097/ACM.0000000000000765

7 The Community as a Classroom: The Invisible Work of Community-Engaged Medical Education

MIRIAM HOFFMAN, CARMELA ROCCHETTI,
MICHAL DIVNEY, AND KIMBERLY BIRDSALL

As one component of our partnership with the medical school, we welcomed an assigned student to work on a community project addressing disparities in preterm birth rates. For part of the project, the medical student participated in a community discussion group with local women. The student arrived eager to learn but soon realized that joining the women's discussion group wasn't going to be as easy as she expected. Despite her high grades, professional dress, and enthusiasm to engage, the women were hesitant to share intimate experiences with this new, visibly nervous young woman. After some time and effort, the lines of communication were opened, resulting in an intimate and honest dialogue.

The student later shared that she was shocked by the level of need and lived experiences of the women. She had studied the determinants of health in the classroom, but here they were brought to life through people like Anna. Anna was a pregnant, unemployed mother-of-two receiving Supplemental Nutrition Assistance Program benefits and other social supports. She was fearful about her health and her pregnancy because she wasn't able to access prenatal care until late in her second trimester. It was difficult to take care of herself and manage her diabetes due to limited transportation and finances. The nearest grocery store was two bus rides away, which forced her to prioritize what she bought based on cost and what she could carry. This experience was powerful for the medical student, who expressed her gratitude for the opportunity to connect directly with community members in such an impactful way.

– Kimberly Birdsall, Executive Director of the
Health Coalition of Passaic County

Any discussion of medical education design should begin by asking *why* we are doing what we are doing. If the purpose of medical education is to develop physicians who are able to care for the well-being of the patients and populations they serve, then the framing of medical education becomes clear. We must think about how we can impact and improve the longevity and well-being of our patients.

Fundamentally, this will take us down a path that may be different from where medical education historically has focused. Rather than starting and ending with the biomedical, to the exclusion of all else, we must include factors such as social context, environment, and behaviour. This is analogous to medicine's increasing focus on addressing social determinants of health in addition to the biologic and other determinants because we know that up to 80 per cent of health outcomes are determined by social and behavioural factors, and only 10–20 per cent by the medical care provided in the healthcare setting.[1,2]

It therefore becomes important to integrate education and training in community health and contextual factors into medical education programs. This can be unchartered territory for many medical educators and curriculum developers. It can be challenging for physicians to seek out or understand this approach, especially if they have a historically narrow view of medical education. In addition, as promulgated in the tenets of community-engaged medical education (CEME), the community must be part of the process, not just the recipient or object of the process.[3]

CEME is complex, requiring the engagement of persons from backgrounds and sectors not historically involved in medical school curriculum development and delivery, and does not lend itself to one cookie-cutter recipe. Rather, there are core principles to guide efforts within each institution. One central tenet is that the persons who develop and run these education programs bring important perspectives and provide critical functions that are required to truly implement a CEME program.[3]

To be successful in this novel approach, medical schools must engage and rely upon the often invisible community engagement specialists. What is a community engagement specialist? This umbrella term represents a broad range of job titles, training, and backgrounds in fields such as public health, social work, psychology, and education, to list only a few. Medical schools and community partners use varied titles for these roles. At the Hackensack Meridian School of Medicine (HMSOM), the community programs team consists of community engagement specialists, community liaisons, and a community programs manager who oversees the department. While there is overlap in these roles and abundant collaboration, each individual has a specialized focus within the team to achieve the goals of CEME.

As illustrated in the introductory vignette, community engagement specialists can also be persons from community organizations who do not work for the medical school but partner with the school to deliver programming for medical students. Community partners come from a wide array of public and private non-profit community-based organizations and other entities who provide needed services in a variety of domains, such as social service agencies, community health centres, schools, municipalities, and more.

In this chapter, we will share perspectives of community-engaged medical educators who have collectively built a robust CEME program – namely, The Human Dimension Program – at the HMSOM in New Jersey, USA. The team includes individuals employed by the school and others who are employed by community agencies who are core partners in the CEME program. They have dedicated their careers to advancing health equity and addressing social determinants of health. Professor Michal Divney LCSW, Human Dimension and Community Programs Manager, brings 20 years of experience in non-profit counselling and expertise in building personalized connections with community members. Kimberly Birdsall MPH, Executive Director of the Health Coalition of Passaic County, has over 25 years of experience in public health and expertise in advancing health equity through diverse partnerships. Dr. Miriam Hoffman, Vice Dean of Academic Affairs and a family physician, and Dr. Carmela Rocchetti, Human Dimension Course Director and an internist, are both physician faculty and administrative leaders at the HMSOM.

We aim to give volume to the voices of the members of this team who are often not front of mind when medical education curriculum development is being discussed. Amplifying and learning from these perspectives is one step towards building medical education training that can create physicians who are able to address *all* of the factors that impact the health outcomes of patients and communities.

Community-Engaged Medical Education: An Academic Perspective

Medical schools across the nation are increasingly recognizing the importance of teaching students how to address the social determinants of health (SDoH).[4,5] SDoH are the non-medical factors that impact an individual's health, such as income, education, food security, and access to care.[6] It is increasingly clear that medical school curricula that include training on racial bias, housing instability, access to care, and other SDoH that reduce healthcare disparities produce physicians who are more likely to practise in underserved communities.[7-9] Medical schools have deployed various types of service learning and community engagement within their curricula, and evidence has shown a benefit for both students and the community.[7] CEME is an effective approach to incorporate SDoH into medical education because it emphasizes the integration and involvement of community-based experiences into medical school curricula and helps students gain a deeper understanding of the social, cultural, and environmental factors that drive health outcomes. Despite the benefits of CEME, implementing it effectively can be challenging as it is complex, resource intensive, and dependent on many variables. As a result, when implemented, CEME is often limited and/or siloed from other aspects of the curriculum.[7,10] As a new medical school with a mission-driven charge, HMSOM embraced a "blank slate" opportunity to develop an entire undergraduate medical education program that was framed by and centred on CEME.

Community-Engaged Medical Education: A Clinical Perspective

As described above, medicine and medical care must focus on all the determinants of health – the different factors that are known to impact health outcomes.[2] Including all the determinants of health in a broad and integrated manner should be incorporated into each medical student's (and physician's) thinking, medical decision-making, and approach to patient care. Just as addressing a patient's social needs cannot be siloed from medical care, medical students need to be trained to cognitively integrate information from all the determinants as they learn content from all the sciences during medical school. This ideally will lead to patient interactions (i.e., history and physical examination) and medical decision-making (e.g, development of assessments and plans) that innately include factors from all the determinants – from the biologic to the social or environmental.

Curricula training students in these areas should include content from the related sciences, but also importantly include experiential activities with community immersion. Powerful experiences like meeting with individuals in their homes or in community centres, observing neighbourhood challenges, and service-learning work can lead to more impactful change in thinking and behaviour than a well-formatted slide deck. Just as medical students integrate content from pharmacology and anatomy into their patient care, the results of these high-impact experiences will be integrated into their patient interactions, medical decision-making, and clinical plan development.

Physicians alone cannot develop and run CEME programs. A CEME curriculum requires partnering with experts from an array of backgrounds, using an integrated and collaborative approach. This will have the added benefit of modelling for our students the interprofessional collaboration that takes place in both clinical and community-based settings. Community engagement specialists are at the heart of this training system.

Community-Engaged Medical Education: Community Engagement Specialists' Perspectives

The key constituents of a medical school are medical students. The educational program exists to serve them and create future physicians. However, for community engagement specialists, there are not one, but two key clients whose needs you are there to meet – medical students and the community. Often, the needs of these two populations are at odds with one another. Students want predictable, structured, time-efficient community immersion experiences that they can learn from and feel good about. However, working with individual community members and organizations can present challenges to these desires. In fact, community-based experiences are often unpredictable, dynamic, and time-intensive. As community engagement specialists, our job is to ensure that we provide students with as much support as possible to foster their community-based learning while ensuring that the community we serve feels they are benefiting from the students' work.

– Michal Divney, Human Dimension and Community
Programs Manager

CEME requires the development of long-lasting institutional partnerships, implementation of community immersion programming, and continuous improvement of programming. The community programs team must be continually engaged in community outreach to learn about the community and its needs so that they can develop and sustain institutional relationships that serve as the foundation for many collaborative initiatives. For example, during a free lunchtime program run by a community-based organization (CBO), our community programs team provided a tabletop presentation on digital health literacy while promoting our student home visiting program. We also actively participate in local health coalitions, attend community meetings and networking sessions, and facilitate connection among community partners. We work within our institution's resources to help meet the needs of the community. For example, we recruited physicians to provide nutrition education for seniors and linked our network's community outreach team of public health nurses to conduct health screening and education for interested community partners.

Leveraging the relationships we have built and nurtured, we identify and ask CBOs to partner with us in our programming. Our process includes an explanation of goals and program parameters and the careful setting of expectations. For example, in order to recruit CBOs to partner with our students for community health projects, we provide both written materials delineating the expectations that CBOs may have of our students (e.g., number of hours, project scope) as well as the expectations of them as partners (e.g., frequency and timing of required meetings with students), and we hold several discussions to ensure a good fit. This can be challenging, as both the students' and community partners' time is limited and restricted to certain times of the day. It can sometimes feel like trying to fit a square peg into a round hole.

The team devotes a great deal of time to administratively support our programs and activities. Safety training is provided to students before they conduct home visits and do other community-based work. Policies and processes must be developed and implemented as well as planning, scheduling, and managing multiple complex projects. Ensuring effective communication between all parties is critical. This requires a lot of coordination and upkeep; this behind-the-scenes work is often invisible.

Beyond logistical support, the community programs team serves as professional role models and consultants to our students, guiding students on how to find and evaluate community resources for the families they are working with. The team helps students negotiate their work with CBOs when expectations are not aligned and supports the students with brainstorming and creative problem-solving. We also provide support to faculty mentors to help them navigate and supervise their students' community work.

Community engagement is an ever-evolving process. We continually seek both formal and informal feedback from our faculty and staff, students, and community partners on the effectiveness and efficiency of our programming from both a content and logistical perspective and make improvements accordingly.

Working with the community is not always predictable and requires the ability to be flexible. Students are often unprepared for things like cancellations or how to balance the goals of their assignments with the real-life individuals they are working with. They can become frustrated and feel like they are wasting their time and can assume our program is not well managed. Initially, they can miss the real-world life lessons they are experiencing as these may not be the structured objectives they set out to learn. However, they are learning that families residing in historically underinvested communities often have many challenges that affect their ability to keep appointments and that partner organizations are often stretched thin and under-resourced. Later in the curriculum, once they have seen the impact of all the determinants of health on community members' lives, students often have an "Aha!" moment – when the pieces connect, they truly understand *why* they were learning this material and completing these activities, and they see the connection to providing the highest-quality patient care.

Community-Engaged Medical Education: A Community Partner's Perspective

During the COVID-19 pandemic, we faced challenges determining a virtual, community-based, meaningful project that our assigned medical students could lead. Ultimately, we connected the students to a grant-funded project with a faith-based organization (FBO) offering an eight-week nutrition and physical fitness curriculum to congregations. Scheduling the sessions was challenging; the FBO wanted evening sessions so its members would attend, while the medical students needed daytime sessions. Eventually they were able to find a workable time, but due to the delay, the program had to be condensed and no longer fulfilled the grant requirements. Despite this, we continued the program to ensure the students gained first-hand experience in individuals' real-life barriers to healthy food access and physical activity.

– Kimberly Birdsall

You don't often think of houses of worship, food pantries, rental assistance agencies, or family success centres as organizations that play a role in medical education, but these types of organizations are critical to the health of individuals and communities and therefore need to be a part of medical education. As a coalition who brings these organizations together, when we were approached to partner with the HMSOM to provide community engagement opportunities for medical students, our answer was an immediate yes. Because when you work to address the health and social needs of vulnerable populations you always say yes. You say yes to every opportunity for collaboration and every opportunity that could result in positive change. The bonus of saying yes to a school of medicine partnership is that not only do you get to increase your organization's community reach and program capacity, you also actively participate in the formation of future physicians by providing tangible, real-life experiences and powerful learnings. As T. Harv Eker has said: "What you hear, you forget; what you see, you remember; what you do, you understand."

Our goal is to provide each student with a positive experience and a well-defined, measurable, and impactful project – but this isn't easy. Organizations who do this work are often small, independent non-profit agencies with limited staff who must manage simultaneous priorities to remain sustainable. Most rely upon private and governmental grant funding which include restrictions on the structure, types, and timelines of projects. In addition, these organizations must manage their organizational infrastructure, board governance, program impact, day-to-day operations, grant applications and reporting, and fundraising efforts. It is a lot to manage but we do our best because the work is important and the collaborations are critical to improve the health of our communities.

This partnership with the school of medicine is an opportunity to positively change the trajectory of healthcare through CEME. The work is not simple. Many of our systems are broken. However, the community partnership experience with the school of medicine shows students the strength of cross-sector collaboration and highlights the power future physicians have to be advocates for change.

Concluding Thoughts

As shared by the voices in this chapter, developing, implementing, and continuously improving community-engaged medical education programs is complex and messy. However, it is critical if we want to train the future physician workforce to be able to address *all* the determinants of health.

While these experiences can be unpredictable and less structured than what medical students might prefer, they teach students problem-solving skills at the micro-, meso-, and macro-system levels. Given the range of community-based settings and experiences as well as the complexity of these programs, a skilled and diverse team of community engagement specialists is needed on both the school and community sides. These partnerships deliver effective educational experiences but also model the interprofessionalism and collaboration needed both in the clinical setting and in truly integrating healthcare with community-based entities.

Listening to and learning from the voices of community engagement specialists is valuable for medical students and physicians. In addition to sharing their wisdom, these professionals ensure that a central tenet of community-engaged work is maintained: letting the community and their articulated needs drive efforts. It therefore also gives voice to the people in the communities that we are serving.

Using the same frameworks utilized for development and implementation, future areas of study will focus on assessing the outcomes of community-engaged medical education programs on the students as well as community-based outcomes. This bridges the realms of outcomes-focused medical education research and health services research. Here as well, community engagement specialists will play an important role, both in the implementation of programs and as key stakeholders and leaders in facilitating program assessment and research.

Medicine and medical education have a history of marginalizing voices not aligned with key loci of power. While the knowledge, perspectives, and skills that community engagement specialists bring to medical education are critical, their voices are often not heard or prioritized given the historic power structures, the primacy of the biomedical, and the dynamic and behind-the-scenes nature of their work. Embracing healthcare's focus on the social determinants of health, community health, and population health can serve as an impetus to bring the perspectives and expertise of community engagement specialists into the process and delivery of medical education. This will train future physicians to be well equipped to impact the longevity and well-being of the communities they serve. The sometimes invisible community engagement specialists play a critical role in this paradigm and educational system.

Additional Reading

Strasser, R., Worley, P., Cristobal, F., Marsh, D.C., Berry, S., Strasser, S., and Ellaway, R. 2015. Putting communities in the driver's seat: the realities of community-engaged medical education. *Academic Medicine*, 90(11), 1466–70. https://doi.org/10.1097/acm .0000000000000765

Committee on Educating Health Professionals to Address the Social Determinants of Health, Board on Global Health, Institute of Medicine, National Academies of Sciences, Engineering, and Medicine. 2016. *A Framework for Educating Health Professionals to Address the Social Determinants of Health* [Internet]. National Academies Press. Available from: www.ncbi.nlm.nih.gov/books/NBK395983/

Schroeder, S.A. 2007. We can do better – improving the health of the American people. *New England Journal of Medicine*, 357(12), 1221–8. https://doi.org/10.1056/nejmsa073350

Rocchetti, C., Duffy, C., Winter, R.O., and Hoffman, M. 2025. Transforming the Ecosystem of Medical Education: Community-Engaged Medical Education (CEME). *Academic Medicine, 100*(9), 1106. https://doi.org/10.1097/ACM.0000000000006050

Rosen, L., and Rocchetti, C. 2025. The human dimension: integrating whole health into a community-engaged medical education curriculum. *Explore.* 22(1), 103302. https://doi.org/10.1016/j.explore .2025.103302.

References

1. Hood, C.M., Gennuso, K.P., Swain, G.R., and Catlin, B.B. 2016. County health rankings: relationships between determinant factors and health outcomes. *American Journal of Preventive Medicine*, 50(2), 129–35. https://doi.org/10.1016/j.amepre.2015.08.024

2. Schroeder, S.A. 2007. We can do better – improving the health of the American people. *New England Journal of Medicine*, 357(12), 1221–8. https://doi.org/10.1056/nejmsa073350

3. Strasser, R., Worley, P., Cristobal, F., Marsh, D.C., Berry, S., Strasser, S., and Ellaway, R. 2015. Putting communities in the driver's seat: the realities of community-engaged medical education. *Academic Medicine*, 90(11), 1466–70. https://doi.org/10.1097/acm.0000000000000765

4. Association of American Medical Colleges (AAMC) and American Medical Association (AMA). 2022. Functions and structure of a medical school: standards for accreditation of medical education programs leading to the MD Degree. [Internet]. Liaison Committee on Medical Education (LCME). Available from: https://lcme.org/publications/

5. AAMCNEWS. 2021. Medical schools overhaul curricula to fight inequities. Available from: www.aamc.org/news-insights/medical-schools-overhaul-curricula-fight-inequities

6. CDC. 2024. Social Determinants of Health. Centers for Disease Control and Prevention. Published January 17, 2024. Available from https://www.cdc.gov/about/priorities/why-is-addressing-sdoh-important.html

7. Arebalos, M.R., Botor, F.L., Simanton, E., and Young, J. 2021. Required longitudinal service-learning and its effects on medical students' attitudes toward the underserved. *Medical Science Educator*, 31(5), 1639–43. https://doi.org/10.1007/s40670-021-01350-7

8. Ko, M., Heslin, K.C., Edelstein, R.A., and Grumbach, K. 2007. The role of medical education in reducing health care disparities: the first ten years of the UCLA/Drew Medical Education Program. *Journal of General Internal Medicine*, 22(5), 625–31. https://doi.org/10.1007/s11606-007-0154-z

9. Rabinowitz, H.K., Diamond, J.J., Markham, F.W., and Wortman, J.R. 2008. Medical school programs to increase the rural physician supply: a systematic review and projected impact of widespread replication. *Academic Medicine*, 83(3), 235–43. https://doi.org/10.1097/ACM.0b013e318163789b

10. Hunt, J.B., Bonham, C., and Jones, L. 2011. Understanding the goals of service learning and community-based medical education: a systematic review. *Academic Medicine*, 86(2), 246–51. https://doi.org/10.1097/ACM.0b013e3182046481

8 The Unseen Role of Licensed Practice Nurses in Medical Students' Workplace Learning

FRANCISCO OLMOS-VEGA, JAZMIN ZULETA-GARCÍA, AND RENATE KAHLKE

I distinctly remember the beginning of my neuro-anaesthesia rotation. I was in the second year of my anaesthesiology residency, and it was my first time doing a rotation with highly complex patients. I was particularly nervous because the rotation teacher was rigorous and demanding. I reviewed the patient's history thoroughly and read about the case we would give the day before. Milena, the licensed practice nurse permanently assigned to all neuro-anaesthesia cases, approached me before the teacher arrived and explained how things worked in the OR [operating room], what things were usually prepared for those cases, and how my teacher liked me to prepare the OR. I felt a mixture of strangeness and gratitude; I could not have done my job so well with all the preparation in the world. It baffled me because I always saw practice nurses as technicians assisting me during my OR practices, not as a source of knowledge, certainly not as trainers; that was my supervisor's role. I never knew if it was something she did with all the residents or if she had noticed my nervousness and then decided to help me selflessly. Until then, I had never been so dependent on the practice nurse and therefore had not recognized their immense role in my training. From then on, I started talking directly to them about preparing each case. It is a favour I will never be able to repay.

– Francisco Olmos-Vega, anaesthetist and assistant professor

Workplace learning constitutes the backbone of medical education. During their clinical rotations, medical learners are expected to acquire the competencies to work as future professionals, develop a distinctive professional identity, and collaborate with various healthcare professionals.[1–3] Their ability to achieve these competencies hinges on integrative experiences within complex healthcare teams. By interacting with other healthcare professionals, medical students learn the skills they will need as future professionals, including finding their place within teams that include a rotating cast of attending surgeons and anaesthetists, other residents at various levels of training, pharmacists, registered nurses, and licensed practical nurses (LPNs).[3]

Navigating this complex network of actors is challenging, particularly when interprofessional hierarchies can inhibit productive working relationships and silence the voices of those perceived as lower in the interprofessional pecking order.[4,5] In medical education, these hierarchies are learned and reinforced when workplace learning emphasizes the role of physician team members, neglecting the pivotal roles of other health professionals.[6] This systematic marginalization and neglect can put student learning and patient care at risk as medical learners struggle to acquire many crucial competencies they need to practise alongside other professionals.[7] In our experience, even when interprofessional education (IPE) occurs, it often focuses on university-educated health professionals who are usually trained at the same institutions, such as registered nurses, pharmacists, and respiratory therapists. In particular, the voices of LPNs are rarely heard since their training occurs in technical colleges, away from more prestigious, university-trained professions. However, their roles are often integral to the successful functioning of many healthcare contexts. This is particularly true of the operating room (OR), where learning and work are demanding and highly dependent on interprofessional collaboration.[8] The OR could only function with the crucial role of the LPN, and, as we will explore in detail below, they are also integrative to the training process of medical learners. In this chapter, we seek to explore the contributions of LPNs in medical education, highlighting the voice of one of our co-authors, an LPN working in the OR in Bogotá, Colombia. Unfortunately, LPNs often remain on the sidelines and are rarely called upon to participate in the education of other professionals or to share their expertise. Furthermore, there hasn't been much exploration in the literature regarding the involvement of technician-level professionals in medical education. Through her story, we explore both how LPNs can contribute to medical education and enhance interprofessional practice, as well as the barriers that prevent LPNs from engaging in IPE. We can only capitalize on the potential of LPNs in medical education if we understand their role and potential – the first step is exploring that contribution and then bringing intention to it.

We write this chapter as a collaborative team of an LPN, an anaesthetist, and a medical education researcher. To centre the voice and stories of LPNs, Jazmin Zuleta-García (an LPN practising in Bogotá, Colombia) shares her experiences and thoughtful reflections about practising as an LPN and working with medical learners. Jazmin's narratives were shared with the team in Spanish. They were translated and summarized into the excerpts that appear in this chapter. Francisco Olmos-Vega, an anaesthetist and assistant professor trained and working in Bogotá, acted as the interviewer, asking Jazmin about her experiences as an LPN working with medical learners. It was essential to the team that Jazmin's experiences serve as the foundation for the chapter; therefore, based on this interview, Francisco created a first draft of the narrative in Spanish and shared it with Jazmin to ensure it adequately represented their conversation and her experiences. After revising the draft to incorporate Jazmin's comments, Francisco translated the narrative into English. Francisco and Renate Kahlke (a PhD-trained medical education researcher) worked together to develop the chapter (in English) and to bring external literature into the manuscript to add evidence-based considerations to it. Francisco conferred with Jazmin regularly to clarify concepts and ensure the chapter matched her expectations and experiences. Francisco also shares his narrative to offer the additional context of a clinician's experience with IPE in the OR and highlight the LPN role in this work. Renate's previous experiences as a manager of an extensive university-based IPE program also informed the work since she drew on the challenges and opportunities she encountered there.

Giving Voice to Licensed Practice Nurses

As in many countries in North America and Europe, practice nurses are a fundamental component of the healthcare system in Colombia. They constitute a large proportion of the healthcare workforce and are responsible for a significant amount of direct patient care. To become a practice nurse, these professionals must acquire a post-secondary education degree equivalent to a bachelor's degree and complete a two-year training program that, in Colombia, is classified as technical training. However, this generic depiction of the LPN role gives us little understanding of how LPNs integrate into care settings – their pivotal role on healthcare teams as choreographers of many administrative and patient-care tasks. In addition, LPNs often have the most direct contact with patients and thus also hold critical knowledge about their patients' histories and preferences. As the following narrative from Jazmin illustrates, sharing that knowledge with residents and medical students is part of how LPNs support medical education, but realizing that sharing isn't straightforward:

My name is Jazmin, and I have been an OR LPN for 10 years. I have also worked in the same hospital for 10 years. Since I have the most direct contact with undergraduate students and residents in the OR, I will relate my specific experiences in that area.

I usually do not know who my staff members will be ahead of time, so I find out once I see the OR schedule. The scheduling specifies the surgeon and anaesthesiologist in charge of the patient. The scrub nurses also follow a specific rotation, so I may know which one I will work with beforehand. Residents are more challenging to predict, and I usually find out with whom I will work that day. The resident I have the most contact with is the anaesthesiology resident. Since we work as a team, I usually ask them directly what they will need for the surgeries scheduled in that room that day. Of course, I could ask their faculty member [staff anaesthesiologist] those same questions. Still, I always prefer to ask the resident first and then corroborate the answer with the anaesthesiologist, as it is an excellent way to integrate the resident into the surgical team, especially if they are starting their residency.

If you ask me, hierarchies are not so marked in surgical suites. I usually think I work with the resident rather than for the resident. I understand they come with evident and structured knowledge and skills; however, I am also aware of all the knowledge I have about how things work in the OR, which they usually do not have. After so many years, I also know anaesthesiologists' tastes and preferences when working on a specific case. Usually, this is the knowledge that I kindly share with the residents, either because they come to me in search of it or because I realize that they may be lost concerning details that, although small, are decisive when integrating into the surgical team. When they share their anaesthetic plan with me, I often recommend how the anaesthesiologist likes to prepare each case, and they generally accept those suggestions. Senior residents may more reluctantly take these suggestions because perhaps they feel they have more experience. Suppose they don't consider my recommendations and face a new attending or a more complex surgery. In that case, they may end up experiencing friction with the anaesthesiologist because they didn't follow my advice. Obviously, I can't force people to abide by my advice, but sooner or later they notice the vital perspective I provide. The contact I have with other residents, such as those in surgical specialties, is scarcer and sporadic. While I also have a broader knowledge of how things work, I generally only share it if they ask me specific or more direct questions.

And not to mention the undergraduate students; I usually feel that they are much more lost in the OR workflow, and I don't feel them as integrated into the surgical team. I often think they are a hindrance in the OR because they are not contributing to the work we have to do and instead can interfere with mine. I would like a more participatory role in their training, such as with the anaesthesiology residents. When I see them more interested, I try to explain to them how things work: where they can find the patients who are going to be operated on, where in the OR they can place themselves to have better visibility

of the surgical field, or who the anaesthesiologist assigned to the room is and how they like their workplace organized. I feel that this helps them integrate into the team and feel useful inside the OR. The ones I don't engage with look like zombies lost without direction. What happens is that at the end of the day, it is not my responsibility and they have their teachers, who are the ones who should make an effort to create value for the time spent by their students in these clinical rotations. It is also important to consider that my job is, first and foremost, LPN in the OR, not a medical teacher. We work in an internationally accredited hospital, so the pressure to provide efficient, high-quality patient care is high. The chief nurses are always on us to complete our duties fast, so the time I have available to guide these students is scarce. That is why I end up prioritizing my tasks over their guidance.
– Jazmin Zuleta-García, licensed practice nurse
[translated from original Spanish by Francisco Olmos-Vega]

As Jazmin describes in the narrative, LPNs carry out many direct patient-care tasks and have a privileged position in knowing "how things work" – she's aware of the systems and people operating in the context, which can change daily. Jazmin's narrative brings forth two underrecognized but pivotal roles that LPNs play in medical education and healthcare practice: they act as choreographers in the OR and they improvise to share their insights with medical learners. Both of these contributions can potentially enhance learners' participation in the OR, even though their learning institutions do not sanction this pedagogical labour. As Jazmin states: "At the end of the day, it [medical education] is not my responsibility."

As choreographers, LPNs play a critical role in ensuring learners can manage staff physicians' preferences, fulfil the tasks required to contribute to a surgery, position themselves in the space of the OR, and integrate within the OR's culture. As Francisco's opening narrative suggests, the privileged knowledge LPNs can share is often overlooked in medical education. The type of contextual knowledge involved in this choreography is rarely recognized – little of it can be learned from books or manuals since the context is ever-evolving and changes as the actors within the context change. Since LPNs' engagement in medical education is unstructured and unsanctioned, this critical knowledge is passed on informally and piecemeal, based on the preferences of the individual LPN and the engagement of individual learners.

Thus, LPNs' participation in medical education is an act of improvisation. Jazmin finds ways to participate in medical education, working from her belief in the power of her knowledge and her desire to support the education of others. However, she must also navigate the constraints of her position in the OR hierarchy – learners may not recognize her knowledge and feel that "they have more experience" – and manage the other tasks she must complete within a busy OR. In a setting with a heavy intraprofessional emphasis on medical education, tensions inevitably arise between her role as a healthcare team member and as a potential guide for medical students. Jazmin's narrative highlights how LPNs often improvise and make individual choices about whether and how to engage with learners. LPNs read the situation, gauge the learners' interest, and decide whether and how they will pass on their knowledge and facilitate integration in the team. For example, Jazmin selectively chooses to engage with residents instead of communicating directly with the attending anaesthesiologist to benefit the learners. In this way, LPNs can act as gatekeepers that could facilitate (or hinder) medical students' participation and, therefore, their learning. This is especially palpable in the difference between Jazmin's engagement with undergraduate and postgraduate students. As postgraduate students have a more prominent role within the healthcare team, LPNs might find it easier to engage with them. Conversely, undergraduate students' ambiguous role in some scenarios, such as the OR, might result in the perception of them being a hindrance to the healthcare team workflow.

Although the role is unsanctioned, LPNs' ability to improvise their participation in medical education shows great promise. Jazmin teaches based on individuals' needs and engagement at the moment, building relationships and enhancing learning within the OR that may not be possible to teach more formally. However, this unsanctioned activity is also uncomfortable. Many learners may not receive vital contextual knowledge because they are perceived as disengaged, and its absence could undermine patient care or even patient safety. At the same time, this unsanctioned activity burdens LPNs, who are already some of the lowest-paid healthcare team members and are also not recognized or compensated when they take on educational tasks in addition to their clinical duties.

Interprofessional Learning at the Workplace

In many healthcare settings, intraprofessional medical education is prioritized over interprofessional learning, relegating the latter to a secondary position.[6] While clinical supervisors are crucial in helping medical students acquire clinical competencies,[9] interprofessional healthcare team members often do not receive the recognition they deserve. Unfortunately, this overemphasis on intraprofessional education has resulted in informal, accidental, and often inconsequential interprofessional interactions for medical students' learning. This highlights the need for more formalized and valued IPE; our discussion above has shown how the contributions of interprofessional healthcare teams can profoundly impact medical students' training. Research on IPE in medical education has shown two overarching roles of healthcare allies in medical students' learning: first, they engage in direct and indirect teaching practices[9] and second, they act as gatekeepers, regulating access to learning opportunities in the workplace.[10] We will discuss these two themes in relation to Jazmin's narrative.

Healthcare allies play an important role in guiding medical students within the workplace. For example, nurses offer valuable advice and feedback to students on communication skills,[11] while pharmacists help develop prescribing competencies.[12] Healthcare allies also help students understand the various roles within the healthcare team and how they work in different contexts.[13] The significance of healthcare allies' guidance is evident in Jazmin's choreography role; as the LPN on the OR team, she chooses to share their expertise, contributing to students' learning and engagement with the entire team. However, students often undervalue this guidance, as described in Francisco's narrative at the beginning of the chapter. Such underplay has been well described with healthcare team members who hold a professional level of training;[9] this undervaluing could be even more pronounced when those team members hold a technician level of training.

In the workplace, healthcare allies also regulate medical students' access to learning opportunities. For instance, nurses may impede students' access to practice opportunities if they perceive them as incompetent or unmotivated.[10] Additionally, the entire healthcare team may not engage with residents who are merely passing through a clinical rotation, which can hinder their transition into new teams.[3] These practices can be viewed as improvisational acts similar to those described by Jazmin. In such situations, healthcare allies exercise their agency to either facilitate or obstruct learning opportunities for medical students. For instance, by neglecting students, an LPN could deprive them of potentially enriching experiences in the OR. Therefore, it is crucial to transform these improvisational acts into more structured and formal interactions that can better facilitate students learning at the workplace. To do this, we must first surpass all the IPE barriers entrenched in the workplace.

These IPE barriers and challenges may reflect broader issues affecting interprofessional collaboration in healthcare. For example, power imbalances and interprofessional friction due to established hierarchies constitute significant threats to interprofessional collaboration success,[14,15] while also hindering interprofessional learning. These hierarchies can be difficult to challenge, as different professions are commonly socialized to perceive themselves as having contrasting attributes; for example, physicians often see themselves as leaders of the healthcare team and nurses as secondary agents with less power or authority.[16] Much of the learning that either reinforces or subverts professional hierarchies occurs in the authentic interprofessional contexts of the workplace. Furthermore, a disproportionate emphasis on intra-professional education has perpetuated professional silos that isolate medical students from healthcare allies.[17] This siloed learning, in turn, further entrenches power imbalances and professional hierarchies,[18,19] since the contributions of those perceived as lower in the hierarchy remain shrouded. As a result, medical learners often develop a partial understanding of healthcare allies' duties and roles,[20,21] which can create misunderstandings in the scope of practice or responsibilities,[20,21] hinder learners' integration into the healthcare team, and lead learners to neglect feedback received from other professions.[18,20]

Concluding Thoughts

Licensed Practice Nurses (LPNs) are crucial in medical education at all levels. They bring unique perspectives and expertise to the learning environment, often improvising and engaging in interprofessional education by guiding students in understanding operating room (OR) choreographies and rhythms. Despite their contribution, this type of learning often remains unstructured and sporadic and is even absent in undergraduate education. To better engage LPNs in medical education, it is important to highlight their voices and contributions. This involves dismantling physicians' overrepresented influence in workplace settings and creating formal mechanisms that empower LPNs to participate in workplace learning. For instance, LPNs' perspectives could be included in the formal curriculum and solicited informally in interprofessional interactions. LPNs' expertise could also be incorporated into assessment processes. Incorporating LPNs in formal and informal learning mechanisms would significantly impact medical education. It would provide a more diverse learning environment and foster interprofessional collaboration. Acknowledging and highlighting LPNs' contributions can also strengthen their professional identity and role within the healthcare team. Engaging LPNs in medical education is crucial in building a more comprehensive, collaborative, and inclusive healthcare system.

Additional Reading

Stalmeijer, R.E. and Varpio, L. 2021. The wolf you feed: challenging intraprofessional workplace-based education norms. *Medical Education*, 55(8), 894–902. https://doi.org/10.1111/medu.14520

Jansen, I., Silkens, M.E.W.M., Galema, G., Vermeulen, H., Geerlings, S.E., Lombarts, K.M.J.M.H., and Stalmeijer, R.E. 2023. Exploring nurses' role in guiding residents' workplace learning: a mixed-method study. *Medical Education*, 57(5), 440–51. https://doi.org/10.1111/medu.14951

Bannister, S.L., Dolson, M.S., Lingard, L., and Keegan, D.A. 2018. Not just trust: factors influencing learners' attempts to perform technical skills on real patients. *Medical Education*, 52(6), 605–19. https://doi.org/10.1111/medu.13522

References

1. Teunissen, P.W. 2015. Experience, trajectories, and reifications: an emerging framework of practice-based learning in healthcare workplaces. *Advances in Health Sciences Education*, 20(4), 843–56. https://doi.org/10.1007/s10459-014-9556-y

2. Monrouxe, L.V. 2010. Identity, identification and medical education: why should we care? *Medical Education*, 44(1), 40–9. https://doi.org/10.1111/j.1365-2923.2009.03440.x

3. Olmos-Vega, F.M., Dolmans, D.H.J.M., Guzmán-Quintero, C., Echeverri-Rodriguez, C., Teunissen, P.W., and Stalmeijer, R.E. 2019. Disentangling residents' engagement with communities of clinical practice in the workplace. *Advances in Health Sciences Education*, 24(3), 459–75. https://doi.org/10.1007/s10459-019-09874-9

4. Bunniss, S., and Kelly, D.R. 2013. Flux, questions, exclusion and compassion: collective learning in secondary care. *Medical Education*, 47(12), 1197–208. https://doi.org/10.1111/medu.12281

5. Gergerich, E., Boland, D., and Scott, M.A. 2019. Hierarchies in interprofessional training. *Journal of Interprofessional Care*, 33(5), 528–35. https://doi.org/10.1080/13561820.2018.1538110

6. Stalmeijer, R.E., and Varpio, L. 2021. The wolf you feed: challenging intraprofessional workplace-based education norms. *Medical Education*, 55(8), 894–902. https://doi.org/10.1111/medu.14520

7. Billett, S.R. 2014. Securing intersubjectivity through interprofessional workplace learning experiences. *Journal of Interprofessional Care*, 28(3), 206–11. https://doi.org/10.3109/13561820.2014.890580

8. Lillebo, B., and Faxvaag, A. 2015. Continuous interprofessional coordination in perioperative work: an exploratory study. *Journal of Interprofessional Care*, 29(2), 125–30. https://doi.org/10.3109/13561820.2014.950724

9. Jansen, I., Silkens, M.E.W.M., Galema, G., Vermeulen, H., Geerlings, S.E., Lombarts, K.M.J.M.H., and Stalmeijer, R.E. 2023. Exploring nurses' role in guiding residents' workplace learning: a mixed-method study. *Medical Education*, 57(5), 440–51. https://doi.org/10.1111/medu.14951

10. Bannister, S.L., Dolson, M.S., Lingard, L., and Keegan, D.A. 2018. Not just trust: factors influencing learners' attempts to perform technical skills on real patients. *Medical Education*, 52(6), 605–19. https://doi.org/10.1111/medu.13522

11. Varpio, L., Bidlake, E., Casimiro, L., Hall, P., Kuziemsky, C., Brajtman, S., and Humphrey-Murto, S. 2014. Resident experiences of informal education: how often, from whom, about what and how. *Medical Education*, 48(12), 1220–34. https://doi.org/10.1111/medu.12549

12. Noble, C., Brazil, V., Teasdale, T., Forbes, M., and Billett, S. 2017. Developing junior doctors' prescribing practices through collaborative practice: sustaining and transforming the practice of communities. *Journal of Interprofessional Care*, 31(2), 263–72. https://doi.org/10.1080/13561820.2016.1254164

13. Rees, C.E., Crampton, P., Kent, F., Brown, T., Hood, K., Leech, M., Newton, J., Storr, M., and Williams, B. 2018. Understanding students' and clinicians' experiences of informal interprofessional workplace learning: an Australian qualitative study. *BMJ Open*, 8(4), e021238. https://doi.org/10.1136/bmjopen-2017-021238

14. Supper, I., Catala, O., Lustman, M., Chemla, C., Bourgueil, Y., and Letrilliart, L. 2014. Interprofessional collaboration in primary health care: a review of facilitators and barriers perceived by involved actors. *Journal of Public Health*, 37(4), 716–27. https://doi.org/10.1093/pubmed/fdu102

15. Xyrichis, A., and Lowton, K. 2008. What fosters or prevents interprofessional teamworking in primary and community care? A literature review. *International Journal of Nursing Studies*, 45(1), 140–53. https://doi.org/10.1016/j.ijnurstu.2007.01.015

16. Nugus, P., Greenfield, D., Travaglia, J., Westbrook, J., and Braithwaite, J. 2010. How and where clinicians exercise power: interprofessional relations in health care. *Social Science & Medicine*, 71(5), 898–909. https://doi.org/10.1016/j.socscimed.2010.05.029

17. Hall, P. 2005. Interprofessional teamwork: professional cultures as barriers. *Journal of Interprofessional Care*, 19(sup1), 188–96. https://doi.org/10.1080/13561820500081745

18. Miles, A., Ginsburg, S., Sibbald, M., Tavares, W., Watling, C., and Stroud, L. 2021. Feedback from health professionals in postgraduate medical

education: influence of interprofessional relationship, identity and power. *Medical Education*, 55(4), 518–29. https://doi.org/10.1111/medu.14426

19. Baker, L., Egan-Lee, E., Martimianakis, M.A.T., and Reeves, S. 2011. Relationships of power: implications for interprofessional education. *Journal of Interprofessional Care*, 25(2), 98–104. https://doi.org/10.3109/13561820.2010.505350

20. Goldman, J., Reeves, S., Wu, R., Silver, I., Macmillan, K., and Kitto, S. 2015. Medical residents and interprofessional interactions in discharge: an ethnographic exploration of factors that affect negotiation. *Journal of General Internal Medicine*, 30(10), 1454–60. https://doi.org/10.1007/s11606-015-3306-6

21. Duin, T.S.V., de Carvalho Filho, M.A., Pype, P.F., Borgmann, S., Olovsson, M.H., Jaarsma, A.D.C., and Versluis, M.A.C. 2021. Junior doctors' experiences with interprofessional collaboration: wandering the landscape. *Medical Education*, 56(4), 418–31. https://doi.org/10.1111/medu.14711

PART TWO

Evidence Assembly

9 Evidence Assembly – Framing Chapter: On Those Who Make Evidence Assembly Happen

KEVIN W. EVA

I feel compelled to start with a disclosure of bald honesty: when asked to write a framing chapter for this book, I agreed purely because I hold its editors in great esteem. With respect to the book's focus, I struggled to understand the point.

It's not that I don't appreciate the efforts of those who conduct "invisible work." Nor do I underestimate how essential they are to the academic enterprise, both in general terms and in relation to making my own work "visible." Rather, my confusion derived from uncertainty regarding what new insights would be gained from a set of essays on a variety of roles that are connected largely by virtue of having email addresses from the same employer.

There are, without a shadow of a doubt, sociological lessons to be learned about power, anthropological lessons to be learned about culture, and psychological lessons to be learned about motivation, among countless other lessons that could be gleaned from studying those who make medical education happen. However, the aim of this book (and the *Evidence Assembly* section for which I write) is not to share new data regarding how to alter practice; nor is it to deepen theoretical perspective on any of those things.

I could get behind the notion that the book is a celebration of work done well, but it would ruin my effort, to be baldly honest, if I glossed over the fact that variability exists in the quality of performance within any group. There is no role (invisible or otherwise) that guarantees competence, let alone exceptionality, so writing about the variety of things individuals do to enable medical education should not assume the work done to be extraordinary.

Clearly this is not the mindset the editors hoped for when contemplating who could contribute to their effort effectively. So, why am I confessing my uncertainty about the book's value? Because the fact that

I grappled with its importance tells you everything you need to know about its importance – without explicit reminders aimed at heightening awareness, it is far too easy to forget to notice the fullness of people required to make medical education work.

Emphasis should be placed on the words "forget to notice" because I think it likely that everyone who reads these words came to them with a pre-existing understanding that medical education involves a *Chorus of Unheard Voices*. That doesn't stop us from forgetting to notice, which in turn leads to forgetting to acknowledge. Doing so is not simply inconsiderate; it is potentially harmful, as evidenced by an experience I had during the early stages of writing this chapter.

Forgetting to Notice

I am one of many who has deliberately tried, throughout my career, to appreciate and acknowledge the support provided by those who do "invisible work." I loathe hierarchy and generally chafe at formality; hence, I should be as aware as anyone of the hardships that impact upon people who work in the shadows of our institutions. Yet recently, there I was at dinner with staff from an institution that shall remain nameless (not to protect anonymity but to emphasize that it could have been any institution), caught off-guard and left heartbroken by tales of burdens borne.

Those to whom I allude are not prone to complain; they do not shy away from hard work; nor would anyone confuse them with individuals who were not up to their tasks. On the contrary, they are some of my favourite colleagues because they possess every quality an employer could hope for – the perfect combination of capability, dedication, ownership, accountability, and ambition wrapped in personas so graceful and friendly that they exude reassurance, effortlessness, and joy. They hold advanced degrees, have risen through the ranks, and have done so while raising lovely families.

That such impressive people could reach their wits' end is not surprising; work is often stressful and I am sure they, like me, would rather feel stretched than bored. I do not want to argue, therefore, that the pressures they were feeling necessarily indicate a broken system (even though any system that risks losing such individuals deserves a good hard look). Rather, what was unsettling to me was that I forgot to notice the strain they were under. I am in relatively regular communication with the people I am describing and I knew they were busy, but the aplomb with which they do their jobs not only makes their work invisible to many, but it makes their struggles invisible as well. The pressure they felt was causing marital strife; it was preventing sleep; it led tears to flow; yet I didn't see it because I forgot to look.

To be clear, there is nothing I could have done to change their particular situation; I am not telling this tale out of regret for action not taken or with a hero complex. In fact, I am not certain intervention would have been welcomed, because the pain in this instance came from the best possible place – when I asked one of them if it was time to look for a new job, it became clear the toll they felt resulted from a passion to see their program succeed. The work might have been invisible to many, but the benefits it enabled were perfectly tangible to them, and what better than to find meaning in the work one does?

Rather, I am telling this tale because it helped me to understand what the editors of this book were telling me all along – that it is so easy to get caught up in one's own work, life, needs, and wants that we require reminders every now and then that prompt us to notice the sacrifices and struggles of those who operate behind the scenes. Many who make medical education happen are not looking for more visibility, but doing invisible work should not equate to being invisible. Sometimes all it takes to keep moving forward is a reminder of the value one brings (as long as the appreciation is offered authentically); other times will require more deliberate reflection and change, but improvements (for the system and the individuals who make it work) can only begin if we remember to notice what and who is behind the scenes.

Those Who Make Evidence Assembly Happen

With all due respect to those who wrote for other sections in this book, there is no better place to highlight the distinction between invisible and visible work than through the evidence assembly activities described in the chapters that follow. The most visible work a university undertakes, I would argue, is its contributions to the world's knowledge. If you disagree, take a look through the archives of your university's newsletters and your region's newspapers and let me know what proportion of them focus upon advances in research relative to educational and institutional developments. Teachers' work is seen (hopefully) internally, but researchers' work is seen and celebrated internationally. As knowledge producers, we have our names highlighted in the permanent archive of academic papers; we give talks in front of large audiences; and we engage with media, among countless other activities that draw attention to ourselves and the university. These activities are both public and easy to count, two features that make our work highly "visible." As a result, they increase the likelihood of becoming even more noticeable through grants, promotions, accolades, and reputation.

Yet, for every individual who gets put in the spotlight for evidence assembly there is indeed a *thunderous chorus* who enable the work to get done. Chapter 10 offers "stories" of program evaluation from the perspective of academics, physicians, and evaluators, highlighting the complex and collaborative effort required to enable continuous quality improvement in our training programs. Chapter 11 uses poetry to frame reflections on what it is like to be a graduate student, a research assistant, and a supervisor of both groups, drawing attention to "silences" in the literature regarding the vital role these groups play and the risks of inequity that surround them. Chapter 12 details how librarians "lend their expertise" to support trainees and practitioners alike to not only find relevant information, but to enable effective building to be done on the world's pre-existing knowledge for the sake of better healthcare. Chapter 13 reminds us that for every great meal, someone is in the kitchen doing the cooking, as the authors detail the exhausting efforts conference organizers make to enable those who are more visible to share their work, to find colleagues who are like-minded (or good debate partners), and to experience the inspiration that maintains fields of study. Finally, Chapter 14 details the tenuous position that ghostwriters of grants face by presenting dilemmas embedded in having to choose between a career or a contract, having to "game eligibility," and having to navigate institutional processes that reinforce their invisibility. I leave it to readers to explore the details in the individual chapters, but I would be remiss to not mention that the list of invisible workers who contribute to evidence assembly (perhaps creating a foundation for the next edition of this book?) also includes human resource officers, peer reviewers, and life partners. As an editor myself, it would be negligent to not also point out the invaluable and almost completely invisible work done by journal staff. They are essential given that the value of assembling evidence is strongly related to the lengths to which it can be shared.

A journal's staff is so invaluable that eight years ago, when the editorial office that had served *Medical Education* for over two decades was restructured to account for staff retirements, I was compelled to announce the change with the somewhat morbid analogy that it felt like I had lost my right hand. Journals are the traditional backbone of academia, enabling scholars to share their efforts and insights. For all the talk of impact factor, however, a great deal of a journal's success is driven by its reputation for mounting fair, rapid, and constructive peer review and publication processes. If a journal is slow, has tedious systems, or causes undue frustration, then word spreads, authors stop submitting their best work, and reviewers become less interested in volunteering, creating a spiral of degradation. At the same time, journals have become less about providing a record of a field's understanding (although that remains central) and more about serving as a hub for connections between ideas, between people, between geographic regions, and between eras. All of that requires strong relationships, which are heavily determined by the quality of interactions with and between journal staff.

The editor generally gets the attention and, fairly, the criticism, but it is the staff working behind the scenes who are the fundamental determinant of success. They create systems that improve the efficiency of submission processes; they help us track, identify and understand the expertise (and community-mindedness) of potential reviewers; they facilitate workflows aimed at increasing the speed with which accepted work gets made public. They liaise between the editors and authors (real and potential), reviewers, and board members in ways that fundamentally influence whether people think positively about the journal or stop engaging with it. They edit podcasts and build websites to market our authors' work and gather data to help us understand how we can improve the experience for our many stakeholders. Yet, journal staff remain invisible to the point that the emails they send often don't even bear their own names.

The individuals with whom I have worked in that capacity, if not a thunderous chorus, have at least made me feel exceptionally privileged to work with a smaller *harmonious choir*. They have shown me first-hand that caring about one's work and recognizing every success as a team success enables the whole to become greater than the sum of its parts. While their work may have been invisible to most, it was felt by all both in terms of the quality of the journal's procedures and output as well as through their immeasurable influence of inspiring enthusiasm, aspiration, and creativity from others. It is only through their effort, spirit, and the environment they created that we have been able to engage in the sort of innovation that builds a community and enables activities well beyond the routine, arduous, treacherous, and sometimes tedious curation of submitted articles.

Lessons from Within

Those observations, combined with my earlier (perhaps overly cynical?) comment about not wanting to assume that everyone who does "invisible work" should be sainted, begs the questions of what makes some invisible workers stand out, in what ways, and at what cost?

Fortunately, the five chapters in this section provide ample food for thought in these regards.

My earlier allusion to the benefits that come from finding meaning and value in one's work were prompted in part by various stories in these chapters, told from the perspective of people who do invisible work, that use words like "love," "privilege," "honour," "caring," "relationships," "connection," and "fulfilment." These words were expressed as means of explaining why so many are willing to "lend their expertise," to serve as "sounding boards," to be "enabling," to act as "allies," and to engage in "advocacy" for others.

While contemplating those words, it is valuable to keep others, expressed by Tom Hanks in *A League of Their Own*, in mind: "If it were easy, everybody would do it." Putting forth the effort required to successfully conduct the work described in this section carried a "significant burden," led to "exhaustion" reminiscent of the people I described in my own tale of "forgetting to notice," could leave people feeling "insecure" and "undervalued," and required trade-offs that could undermine "legitimacy" and induce perfectly rational behaviour that carries "risk" of being deemed unethical.

Such challenges draw attention to the poignant words of Finn et al. (Chapter 11): "it can be hard to distinguish where opportunity ends and exploitation starts." Spoken in relation to students feeling compelled to stand out in the competitive environments of academia and medicine, the claim is no less suited to consideration of any of the roles that fall into the category of "invisible" work. When our systems, reward structures, and incentivization schemes require people to choose between economic and symbolic capital, as compellingly argued by Torti et al. (Chapter 14), we must worry about reinforcing a status quo that generates privilege for some and dismisses the lack of advantage to others by claiming it simply to be the way "the game is played."

I urge everyone, as a result, to read the entirety of this book with such concerns in mind because the risk of celebrating the under-appreciated is becoming comfortable with their plight. Every treatment has a side effect, in other words, requiring us to notice that acknowledging those whose work is often invisible risks leaving us feeling content and satisfied that coins of social capital are sufficient to pay for bills of physical or emotional burden. While I said earlier that improvements can only begin if we remember to notice what and who is behind the scenes, taking the next step towards actually improving work for those described is the important follow-on.

I don't claim any magical insight regarding what that next step should be because the challenges are complex, requiring distinct consideration of the particulars of each invisible worker's situation. Again, however, I direct attention to the themes inherent in the chapters on evidence assembly that are included in this section and the insights they provoke. When talking about the benefits and joys experienced by those doing invisible work, it is noticeable that each chapter, in one way or another, talks about the role of community. Whether described as "teamwork," "accountability," "integration," "relationships," "social identities," "diversity," "allyship," or "legitimacy," one cannot help but sense that wellness when doing work is derived from a sense of belonging to something greater than ourselves; from feeling like our work has purpose by virtue of bettering the activities, experiences, or successes of others.

Having managed to notice that, I feel like I have finally come to understand what this book is about: by drawing together the stories it contains we are not only more likely to see the forest for the trees, hear the voices that form the choir, and notice the characters that make up the ensemble, but we may have a means of helping each member in the collective to appreciate that medical education is bigger than any one of us – that it is a means through which countless people leave the world in a better place. With that in mind, I encourage each reader to take a moment to remember to notice someone who is behind the scenes yet plays a vital role in making evidence assembly happen. Then ask yourself what you can do, large or small, to make their world better.

10 The Many Faces of Program Evaluation

KIRANJIT K. BRAR, ADAM HAIN, NEIL GESUNDHEIT, AND STEFANIE S. SEBOK-SYER

In medical education, program evaluation is represented by two separate yet equally important groups: the evaluators, who systematically collect, analyse, and use data to examine the effectiveness and efficiency of programs,[1] and the instructional designers, who apply theory and standards to the design of instructional materials and adapt various aspects within programs over time to facilitate learning.[2] This chapter represents their stories.

> *I hope that people recognize how critical our evaluation team is in terms of their contributions, because oftentimes the evaluation team may be invisible to other groups [faculty, students, patients], but they're a critical part of our curriculum meetings and course debrief meetings, and we include [evaluation data] in all our continuous quality improvement efforts.*
>
> – Preetha Basaviah, Clinical Professor of Medicine

In our data-driven world filled with artificial intelligence and machine learning, the people who collect, analyse, and interpret the data can sometimes fade into the background as we prioritize data. In program evaluation specifically, this makes the people and teams that do evaluation work in medical education appear invisible. In an effort to highlight these individuals, often hidden in plain sight, the authors spoke with eight different members from Stanford University School of Medicine who facilitate program evaluation as a component of their daily work. We present the academic perspectives (Irina Russell, Stefanie Sebok-Syer) to illustrate how program evaluation is incorporated into medical education, the physician-educator perspectives (Preetha Basaviah, Italo Brown, Neil Gesundheit, Tracy Rydel, Georgia Moody) to highlight how program evaluation is incorporated into medical education, and finally the program evaluator perspectives (Kiranjit Brar, Adam Hain) to showcase how iterative improvement cycles are supported using data and program evaluation. Each of these individuals holds multiple roles within medical education, which highlights the integrated nature of their different responsibilities. Although such interrelatedness may mask an inherent complexity and drive invisibility, we believe their rich lived experiences offer a meaningful lens to view program evaluation within medical education as a whole. For instance, when asked to describe their role, one highlighted this complexity:

> *My role is a bit multifaceted. If you imagine a Venn diagram, it definitely overlaps a lot with the evaluation team in terms of support and especially consultation around data, architecture, and presentation. And getting our data out there in an automated, cohesive way, so that evaluation data that's presented is consistent [...] I work a lot with assessments, which overlap with program evaluation of courses in a lot of medical schools [...] my work also really overlaps with a lot of our accreditation requirements [...] And sometimes I negotiate contracts. Sometimes I interview vendors, so that actually does overlap with program evaluation work.*
> – Irina Russell, Director of Education Analytics

The Liaison Committee on Medical Education (LCME), educational decision-makers, stakeholders (i.e., anyone affected by a program or program evaluation), and members of the general public have a vested interest in ensuring that Doctor of Medicine (MD) programs are meeting an established set of standards. Program evaluation is critical to assuring that MD programs are graduating competent individuals who can provide quality care and meet the needs of patients in society. We have all heard the term, and many of us may have even dabbled or lightly participated in some sort of program evaluation, but how often do we consider who is behind this activity? Spoiler alert: there is no omnipotent, omniscient program evaluator who resides in each and every medical school throughout the country. Rather, there are teams of individuals who work collaboratively, and often behind the scenes, to wrangle data and engage in the process of evaluation.

The Program Evaluation Context at Stanford University School of Medicine

The MD program at Stanford University offers a flexible curriculum that includes opportunities to pursue dual degrees, self-directed learning and scholarship, delivered to a relatively small class size of approximately 90 students per year.[3] In 2003–2004, Stanford University School of Medicine underwent a major curriculum change, which resulted in the creation of a dedicated evaluation team.[4] After undergoing another major curriculum revision in 2017–2018, the evaluation team expanded to include instructional development as part of the evaluation cycle to support institutional goals for continuous quality improvement within the curriculum:

> *I was the first person in my role in instructional development. Previously, the evaluation department wasn't doing any instructional development. So, this role was added with the intention of providing a loop to respond to the evaluation data that was coming in from the students. It was intended to provide an opportunity to do some of the things that the students are suggesting in a way that is research-based around educational theory. So, they brought in a person with an instructional design background to gather and look at the evaluation data for a particular course, program, or set of courses, and look at it globally, and respond to that in the way that is most efficient across a number of courses."*
>
> – Adam Hain, Associate Director of Instructional Development

Using Stanford University School of Medicine's MD Program as an example, we foreground the faces of the many individuals (rather than the data they work with) who contribute to program evaluation. We also showcase why the sometimes invisible work of program evaluation is integral to supporting the education of current and future physicians.

Program Evaluation: Academic Perspectives

> *Continuous improvement is better than delayed perfection*
>
> – Mark Twain

Michael Scriven, a pioneer in the field, once described evaluation as a young discipline that is very old in practice.[5] Evaluation has been used for thousands of years and endures today as an important form of inquiry in many disciplines, including medical education.[6] Within the medical education community, however, we lack a shared understanding of the relationship between evaluation and other processes, such as research. This is problematic given how much of our program evaluation theory and methodology overlaps with the social sciences.[7] Even among professionals engaged in program evaluation, the distinction is not always clear:

> *I had no idea how broad the scope of program evaluation in medical education was when I first entered the field. I come from a research background, and I also really*

just enjoy processes and systems. So that's kind of how I ended up in program evaluation – from more of a research and systems perspective. However, program evaluation is not research. That's something that I've learned along the way. They are two distinct disciplines, but there is a little bit of crossover that can happen in service of each.

> – Kiranjit Brar, Director of Evaluation and Instructional Development

Glass and Ellett once stated: "Evaluation – more than any science – is what people say it is; and people currently are saying it is many different things."[8] [(p. 211)] Over 40 years later, this statement is still true, but why? The historical development of program evaluation has undergone several paradigm shifts since its first documented account in 1792.[9] Given the relationship between the broader field of education and medical education, it is not surprising that we have also experienced paradigm shifts around what constitutes program evaluation. Although there are many different approaches to program evaluation, each has been largely influenced by these important paradigm shifts. Program evaluation, specifically in medical education, initially used improvement-oriented approaches such as Patton's[10] utilization-focused evaluation that could inform decision-making.[11] From there, we moved into a theory-driven paradigm where scholars[12] stressed the importance of understanding the assumptions made by stakeholders in order to illuminate a program theory. Where we are now is yet another paradigm that embraces emergence and complexity[11] by using approaches such as systems engineering[13] and guiding principles.[14]

This historical framing is important as we consider not only the work of evaluation teams, but also the principles and standards that influence their approach to scientific inquiry. Yarbrough and colleagues[15] put forth 30 program evaluation standards, organized into five groups: utility, feasibility, propriety, accuracy, and accountability to guide evaluation practice. Within medical education specifically, many of these standards are foundational in the work of evaluators: *"tracking and documentation, and making sure that we are accountable to ourselves in terms of where [data are], and that we have accurate information"* (Irina Russell). However, this emphasis on data and standards can cast a shadow on the individuals that give meaning to these data. Further, given that modern evaluation tends to encompass complex and integrated systems, we need to move beyond focusing on static principles and standards and evolve our thinking to consider the dynamic complexity and emergence that is created when people interact with data. Data are never simply data, and trained individuals such as program evaluators often help ensure that these data are used appropriately:

As someone formally trained in both research and program evaluation, I often find myself straddling the line between using data to support new, generalizable knowledge and to inform the improvement of individuals, programs, and systems. Evaluation and research are different: they are different ways of thinking, they serve different purposes, and they require me to approach and present data differently.

– Stefanie Sebok-Syer, Assistant Professor of Emergency Medicine

With this perspective in mind, it is important to remember that the purpose of program evaluation is to make visible, through interpretations of data, the story about what is happening within a program. The role of an evaluator is to review and interpret data so that it can be presented to stakeholders who absorb and use it to inform future efforts and decision-making. While some may believe that "the data" are telling a story, really it is the evaluator's presentation of the data that allows the story to unfold. And while the process might seem opaque, there is an invisible push from program evaluators that is then amplified by those who steward the data.

Program Evaluation: Physician-Educator Perspectives

The roles and responsibilities of running a medical school are not thrust upon a single individual, likely because of the sheer amount of work required. Program evaluation represents a large part of that work, and it takes a team-based approach to do evaluation well. There are many aspects to consider regarding the continuity of how we teach and have trainees learn medicine. At the forefront, physician leaders believe it is important to work collaboratively to *"ensure that our MD students have a great education, one that transmits the most up-to-date principles of scientific medicine"* (Neil Gesundheit, Senior Associate Dean for Medical Education) and make sure *"what happens in the preclinical space is logically tied to what happens in the clinical space"* (Tracy Rydel, Clinical Professor of Medicine).

As these perspectives highlight, program evaluation is a broad-reaching undertaking that requires a team-based approach to carry out well. The people who are part of these teams, who do this work, are keenly aware of the important contribution they make to medical education:

It is both a privilege and incredible honour to be part of their [students'] journey, and to have this actual quantifiable impact as well as the anecdotal impact of

feeling inspired to train the next generation and give back to a profession that really provided and instilled in me skills, values, and attitudes to help me be successful and thrive. And I think that promise of being able to be there for others, and being able to create systems allows for accessible, consistent education.

– Preetha Basaviah

All of the stakeholders who talked about their program evaluation work wanted others to know that: 1) *"there are lots of people who've been doing this work and pushing the needle forward"* (Italo Brown); 2) *"faculty invest themselves tremendously in creating curricula and in delivering it effectively"* (Neil Gesundheit); 3) *"we put a lot of consideration into the different options and thinking about all perspectives of the students"* (Georgia Moody); and 4) *"we are trying so hard, there's many different stakeholders, we hear you, and we're listening"* (Tracy Rydel).

Regarding the impact of program evaluation in medical education, the humanistic aspect of "putting patients (human beings) at the center of focus; promoting better understanding of the human experiences of both patients and clinicians"[16 (p. 1075)] could not be greater emphasized in these physician's stories. So, as we illustrate later, when *"the data that we were seeing on our national surveys, for instance, showed that our students were not feeling well prepared to care for patients from different backgrounds"* (Kiranjit Brar), it was a call to action. This foregrounding of data can mask the program evaluators that work hard to continually integrate human-centred curricula and the physician-educators who use these data to inform program delivery.

Program Evaluation: Program Evaluator Perspectives

The evaluation team is responsible for bringing together data from internal and external sources to support the continuous quality improvement of the curriculum, while also meeting accreditation expectations. This can be difficult in practice; our work is often quiet and happens behind the scenes, which may cause people to forget we exist sometimes. This is where our instructional development arm helps bring program evaluation to the forefront by creating a cycle of reviewing feedback with stakeholders.

– Kiranjit Brar

The iterative evaluation cycle is often invisible from those not directly involved, partly because we tend to focus on outcomes and data rather than how those things came into existence. The team we outlined above works collaboratively in the service of continuous quality improvement, and while the process is transparent, individuals' contributions to the process may not be as visible. We describe a broad team as part of our evaluation cycle, but there are subsets of evaluators that lead different parts of the cycle. At our institution, the collection and analysis of program data using student surveys and focus groups are used to engage course faculty who are then offered instructional development support to implement changes. This provides a framework for a continuous quality improvement cycle that allows faculty to innovate their courses, evaluate changes, review feedback, and repeat. However, in between each of these steps are those invisible evaluators who help steward the data and use it to support improvement efforts. This may include introducing faculty development opportunities, finding resources for curricular innovation, or providing feedback on specific course sessions: *"So I help bring forth a data-driven kind of picture of what's happening, whether it's involved with curriculum or it's kind of integrating and tying together curriculum data with teaching and performance outcomes"* (Irina Russell). These iterations and transitions involve invisible work from those in program evaluator roles.

At Stanford, *"every course in the MD program gets evaluated, and that data goes through our department and gets collected and analysed by the evaluation team"* (Adam Hain). We approach evaluating courses in the preclinical and clinical phases of the MD program using the "empowerment evaluation" framework,[4] which is a collaborative approach to program evaluation that engages stakeholders at all levels (students, faculty, evaluators, administrators) as part of the process. And as one evaluator noted *"providing the evaluation data within this structure of support fosters innovation and helps faculty continue to iterate, knowing that they have a partnership with us and will receive useful feedback to help keep things moving; their efforts were seen, recognized, and not invisible"* (Kiranjit Brar). In this way, the empowerment process generates visibility for all stakeholders.

Program evaluation in medical education is complex *"because of the underlying crossover with accreditation requirements that is often driving evaluation work"* (Kiranjit Brar). Our evaluators highlighted that the LCME plays an important role in how program evaluation is conducted within medical education. Data necessary for accreditation are collected not only within the institution, but additional data sources also supplement undergraduate medical education program evaluation by providing national benchmarks. Program evaluators aid in the interpretation of all these data, which in turn helps guide curricular changes. These data are powerful. As one medical student noted, *"I think we're very fortunate in that the administration is very open to working together with us to create change"* (Georgia Moody, Senior Medical Student, Stanford School of Medicine).

The Social Justice and Health Equity Curriculum: Evaluation in Action*

We conclude this chapter with an example of "program evaluation in action" using a new curricular thread on social justice and health equity created within the Stanford University MD program. Through continuous quality improvement, *"that touches basically on every facet of the medical school"* (Irina Russell), we find ourselves making another major change: developing and implementing a social justice and health equity curriculum in order to support MD students meet the needs of individual patients and society as a whole. We share this example to highlight the cyclical processes of program evaluation, often running invisibly in the background; it is an ideal case demonstrating how an integrated and highly collaborative team moves from feedback to curricular change.

The implementation of the social justice and health equity curriculum thread illustrates how data, collected and interpreted through the work of program evaluators, led to the development of a new curriculum. In addition to program evaluation data, cultural shifts relating to social justice and equity had a notable impact on the medical education community, from the Association of American Medical Colleges to individual medical schools.[17–19] In response, many medical schools began developing curricula aimed at social determinants of health, anti-racism, critical race theory, and health equity:

> *Students had voiced to various faculty members that they wanted to have more understanding of social justice and health equity concepts [...] which revealed a blind spot in their medical education, as they were hearing that there were other [medical school] programs that had curricula devoted to understanding health equity and social justice.*
> — Italo Brown, Assistant Professor of Emergency Medicine

At our institution, it was noted *"that we didn't have enough of a focus on social justice and equity in our previous curriculum"* (Georgia Moody). The work of program evaluators was instrumental in catalysing a change. Based on data, we formed a curriculum subcommittee to support the implementation of the social justice and health equity thread throughout the MD program curriculum. This committee included program evaluators and was tasked with developing new program competencies

---

* The US political climate has shifted since our initial writing of this chapter. Some contextual details have therefore changed.

and longitudinal thread objectives, as well as oversight of the integration of content throughout the curriculum.

Student evaluations were collected at the close of each pre-clerkship course or clerkship period by the program evaluators who collated these data and developed recommendations. Based on evaluation feedback from initial pilots, curricular changes were implemented and re-evaluated iteratively. As we embarked on developing, implementing, and evaluating this new curriculum, the social justice and health equity thread lead reminded us: *"there are no shortcuts [...] you can't see these opportunities and try to fast-track things"* (Italo Brown).

Instead of simply forwarding feedback and suggestions to individual course directors, the social justice and health equity thread integration team met with course directors individually to review the evaluation data and encourage the development of reflective faculty practitioners, based on the framework of empowerment evaluation.[4] These brainstorming sessions were intended to facilitate idea generation around social justice and health equity topics in the context of each organ block or specialty. While the work of program evaluators is often invisible, it was possible to foreground them and their work by including them as members of the social justice and health equity committee. This allowed the program evaluators to leverage instructional development opportunities to become more visible in the process of continuously improving curriculum.

As the social justice and health equity thread continued to develop, student feedback became the primary driver of change, encouraging course directors to continue brainstorming about how to integrate social justice and health equity content into their course. The program evaluators continued to provide support in the background by reviewing data globally across the curriculum to identify opportunities and curricular gaps. This information was then fed back by the evaluators to stakeholders as part of the iterative cycle of implementing curricular thread and since *"in this process you're going to change, you have to. You have to embrace that because it's not just as simple as saying, oh, we would want to, you know, try something that's novel, that's very concrete and hasn't been done before. Now this is all new stuff. This is cutting edge"* (Italo Brown), and our evaluators were there every step of the way guiding the process.

Concluding Thoughts

In summary, we highlight the invisibility of many individual program evaluators that support and contribute to the process of evaluating policies, procedures, and outcomes within MD programs. Medical education is complex, regulated, and dynamic, which often requires a collaborative effort to streamline curriculum, enhance the quality of faculty teaching, and elevate students' learning. So, the next time you are presented with program evaluation data in medical education, consider these invisible trailblazers that work tirelessly to translate information in order to ensure that future doctors have the educational background required to provide excellent patient care.

Additional Reading

Balmer, D.F., Riddle, J.M., and Simpson, D. 2020. Program evaluation: getting started and standards. *Journal of Graduate Medical Education*, 12(3), 345–6. https://doi.org/10.4300/JGME-D-20-00265.1

Patton, M.Q. 2010. *Developmental Evaluation: Applying Complexity Concepts to Enhance Innovation and Use*. Guilford Press.

Yarbrough, D.B., Shulha, L.M., Hopson, R.K., and Caruthers, F.A. 2010. *The Program Evaluation Standards: A Guide for Evaluators and Evaluation Users*. Sage Publications.

References

1. CDC Approach to Program Evaluation. 2024. Available from: https://www.cdc.gov/evaluation/php/about/?CDC_AAref_Val=https://www.cdc.gov/evaluation/index.htm

2. Stes, A., Min-Leliveld, M., Gijbels, D., and Van Petegem, P. 2010. The impact of instructional development in higher education: the state-of-the-art of the research. *Educational Research Review*, 5(1), 25–49. https://doi.org/10.1016/j.edurev.2009.07.001

3. Stanford University – Stanford Medicine – MD program. 2023. Available from: https://med.stanford.edu/md.html

4. Fetterman, D.M., Deitz, J., and Gesundheit, N. 2010. Empowerment evaluation: a collaborative approach to evaluating and transforming a medical school curriculum. *Academic Medicine*, 85(5), 813–20. https://doi.org/10.1097/ACM.0b013e3181d74269

5. Scriven, M. 1996. The theory behind practical evaluation. *Evaluation*, 2(4), 393–404. https://doi.org/10.1177/135638909600200403

6. Onyura, B. 2020. Useful to whom? Evaluation utilisation theory and boundaries for programme evaluation scope. *Medical Education*, 54(12):1100–8. https://doi.org/10.1111/medu.14281

7. Wanzer, D.L. 2021. What is evaluation? Perspectives of how evaluation differs (or not) from research. *American Journal of Evaluation*, 42(1), 28–46. https://doi.org/10.1177/1098214020920710

8. Glass, G.V., and Ellett, F.S., Jr. 1980. Evaluation research. *Annual Review of Psychology*, 31(1), 211–28. https://doi.org/10.1146/annurev.ps.31.020180.001235

9. Hogan, R.L. 2007. The historical development of program evaluation: exploring past and present. *Online Journal for Workforce Education and Development*, 2(4), 5.

10. Patton, M.Q. 2008. *Utilization-Focused Evaluation.* Sage Publications.

11. Haji, F., Morin, M.P., and Parker, K. 2013. Rethinking programme evaluation in health professions education: beyond "did it work?" *Medical Education*, 47(4), 342–51. https://doi.org/10.1111/medu.12091

12. Chen, H.T. 2014. *Practical program evaluation: Theory-Driven Evaluation and the Integrated Evaluation Perspective.* Sage Publications.

13. Rojas, D., Grierson, L., Mylopoulos, M., Trbovich, P., Bagli, D., and Brydges, R. 2018. How can systems engineering inform the methods of programme evaluation in health professions education? *Medial Education*, 52(4), 364–75. https://doi.org/10.1111/medu.13460

14. Balmer, D.F., Anderson, H., and West, D.C. 2023. Program evaluation in health professions education: an innovative approach guided by principles. *Academic Medicine*, 98(2), 204–8. https://doi.org/10.1097/ACM.0000000000005009

15. Yarbrough, D.B., Shulha, L.M., Hopson, R.K., and Caruthers, F.A. 2010. *The Program Evaluation Standards: A Guide for Evaluators and Evaluation Users.* Sage Publications.

16. Thibault, G.E. 2019. Humanism in medicine: what does it mean and why is it more important than ever? *Academic Medicine*, 94(8), 1074–7. https://doi.org/10.1097/ACM.0000000000002796

17. Boatright, D., Berg, D., and Genao, I. 2021. A roadmap for diversity in medicine during the age of COVID-19 and George Floyd. *Journal of General Internal Medicine*, 36, 1089–91. https://doi.org/10.1007/s11606-020-06430-9

18. Brown, A., Auguste, E., Omobhude, F., Bakana, N., and Sukhera, J. 2022. Symbolic solidarity or virtue signaling? A critical discourse analysis of the public statements released by academic medical organizations in the wake of the killing of George Floyd. *Academic Medicine*, 97(6), 867–75. https://doi.org/10.1097/ACM.0000000000004597

19. Lim, G.H.T., Sibanda, Z., Erhabor, J., Bandyopadhyay, S., Neurology and Neurosurgery Interest Group. 2021. Students' perceptions on race in medical education and healthcare. *Perspectives on Medical Education*, 10(2), 130–4. https://doi.org/10.1007/s40037-020-00645-6

11 Research Assistants, Graduate Teaching Assistants, and Graduate Students: A Hidden Force of Research Power within Medical Education

GABRIELLE M. FINN, MEGAN E.L. BROWN, AND CRISTINA COSTACHE

It can be challenging to occupy a hidden and undervalued role. Graduate students, including graduate teaching assistants, and research assistants within medical education meet these criteria. It can also be challenging to know how to supervise those occupying these roles. In this chapter, we outline what is known about the roles, responsibilities, impact, and needs of graduate students, research assistants, and their supervisors. We blend (limited) insights from the academic literature with our personal experiences as graduate students, research assistants, and supervisors in a series of narratives and poems we have written. In doing so, we seek to reveal the hidden depth and power of these roles and illuminate critical areas for future research and exploration.

What Do We Mean by Graduate Students and Research Assistants?

Graduate students are students who, having completed an undergraduate degree, are pursuing academic or professional degrees, certificates, diplomas, or other qualifications (e.g., master's or doctoral (PhD) students).[1] Typically, graduate students study, teach, or conduct research in accordance with the requirements of their degree program. Within some countries, such as the USA, doctoral students are reclassified as doctoral candidates once they pass certain progression milestones and are closer to thesis submission. In other countries, such as they UK, there is no distinction.

Despite most international institutions undertaking research activity, the terminology utilized to describe the academic roles is not universal. One such term is "RA." In some institutions, RA is an abbreviation for a "research associate," or the equivalent of a postdoctoral researcher who is employed to facilitate a research project, often under the guidance of the principal investigator, but they can work independently. Other institutions utilize RA as an abbreviation for the "research assistant" role. Typically, a research assistant is employed to assist with the research process on a specific project, under supervision. A research assistant usually holds a bachelor's degree, or sometimes a master's degree. The research assistant has a low level of autonomy due to the junior nature of the position. Often, people undertake research assistant roles in order to build experience for applications for competitive doctoral programs.

For the remainder of this chapter we will distinguish between research associate and research assistant, using RA to refer to the research assistant role.

Another important junior role is that of the graduate teaching assistant (GTA).[1] A GTA is a paid role within a university for doctoral students who assume extra responsibilities within their department. GTAs often teach, mark, supervise projects, and sometimes assist with research projects other than their own. Literature notes the "ambiguous niche" GTAs hold through their simultaneous roles as teachers, researchers, students, and employees – highlighting the tensions emerging through the conflicting rights and responsibilities associated with such roles.[2] Some institutions build a GTA post into a PhD offering, providing four years of funding instead of three to enable the student to commit to the additional teaching load. The GTA position is useful for postgraduate students seeking academic careers, particularly on teaching and scholarship contracts, as it enables them to gain significant teaching experience and build a portfolio of evidence. Often, institutions will offer a recognized teaching qualification as part of the GTA package. GTAs have their fees paid and receive a stipend. As a condition of this, they are often required to do a minimum number of hours of teaching, with the option to take on extra hours on an hourly rate of pay. However, some institutions will enable students to work whatever number of hours fits their capacity. Globally, terminology and responsibilities may differ. For example, some countries refer to GTA positions as graduate assistantships, but the role may be assisting with research instead of, or as well as, teaching.

It is worth noting that there are often issues with power imbalance and autonomy for RAs and GTAs. Saying no to work that may not align with the graduate student's interests or may be excessive in terms of workload can be troublesome, especially if the GTA's management falls to their doctoral supervisor. They often can feel overworked and undervalued, despite their documented contributions to driving research, academic entrepreneurship, and teaching.[2,3]

This chapter shares the lived experiences of the three authors, as graduate students, research assistants, and supervisors. Megan recently completed her PhD after giving up clinical practice. Cristina is a doctor working internationally who is also working as a research assistant and transitioning to become a graduate student. Gabrielle has supervised both Megan and Cristina, as well as having worked as a research assistant herself.

What Is It Like to Be a Graduate Student?

There is no singular experience of graduate studies, though commonalities across experiences do exist. Here, Megan reflects on the highs and lows of her experiences as a graduate (PhD) student. As we will explore below, this burden may be particularly troubling in the face of ambiguity on the role, responsibilities, and needs of graduate students.

I came straight to my PhD from clinical practice, in the knowledge that I was leaving clinical practice for academia (for many reasons including frustration with working conditions in the UK as a neurodivergent individual). Mostly, I loved my PhD, but it wasn't without its ups and downs.

In total, my studies took me four years full-time, which, although not unusual, is a substantial commitment within which life can change significantly. And for me it did – I had two children and so two maternity leaves during my PhD, got married, became disabled, and (what's more), from my second year onwards, studied during COVID-19. In many ways, it was a heavy lift. I am lucky that my PhD was funded, but with the addition of children to our lives, I needed to work in addition to my studies part-time throughout the course of my PhD, which at times was challenging to balance alongside my thesis and family commitments. I have a tendency to say "yes" to every opportunity (many academics I know share this toxic trait).

I am privileged to be well supported personally, with a fantastic network of friends and family close by. My primary supervisor (who so happens to be a co-author on this chapter!) was an incredible source of support in the face of major life events, academic hurdles, and trying to forge a career within medical education. I have also been fortunate to find connections with researchers in medical education through my supervisor and academic events that have helped me find meaning in this field and friendship with colleagues. I can't overstate how important this has been. Throughout my PhD, I felt and experienced the stigma that those working in medical education often encounter. I had well-respected clinicians scoff at the value of medical education research and tell me directly that I could not have a career in the field if I was not willing to return to clinical practice.

Overall, I have made lifelong friends in medical education and am lucky enough to work with them on many projects still. I mostly feel like I am working upstream and trying to change education and training for the benefit of learners and patients, which is incredibly fulfilling. I have to admit I didn't really know what I was letting myself in for at the start of my PhD and got lucky with my supervisor. I have seen others be less fortunate, with negative consequences. The stigma in medical education regarding the legitimacy of a person's background and input and the precarious nature of academic employment (and the disproportionate negative impact on those with minoritized identities) are structural issues that have been significant negatives within my experience. We should all be working to change the structures of academic employment and the culture within these structures.

– Megan E.L. Brown Senior Research Associate

Megan's poem (Figure 11.1) considers the mental toll that PhD studies can take and the challenge of persisting in the face of such a burden. As we will explore below, we see this burden as particularly troubling in the face of a lack of guidance on the role, responsibilities, and needs of graduate students.

There is little empirical evidence, unfortunately, which documents the unique contributions and merit of graduate students. In his 2009 study in the Netherlands, ten Cate notes a rapid increase in the number of PhD students within medical education between 1999 and 2009, with 66 medical education PhD students active in the country in 2009.[4] The focus of ten Cate's study is unique, and, to our knowledge, has not been replicated in other countries where the field of medical education is well established. Not only is there a relative paucity of work documenting the numbers of graduate students working within medical education, but there is little research on their experience – including their training needs, career development needs and support, and career paths and destinations. Most literature published on the topic of graduate students is done from the perspective of students themselves. There are, for example, useful tips-based articles on completing medical education PhDs or doctoral studies.[5] While they are a fantastic resource for prospective and new students, these articles are descriptive and experience-based (in a way, like the poems we have showcased) rather than representing organized empirical research on the roles, responsibilities, and experiences of students. Without formal, empirical exploration it is difficult to appreciate graduate student experiences and needs across the spectrum of institutions offering postgraduate medical education qualifications. Making recommendations regarding enhancing the role and support are, therefore, challenging.

Within academic medicine literature more broadly, PhD students and their contributions are more visible. Combined MD/PhD programs are well established at several institutions, and there seems to be a greater understanding in the literature regarding the needs and contributions of students studying on these programs.[6] Recent research within medical education suggests that there is a hierarchy within medical education careers, where clinical researchers are able to access opportunities

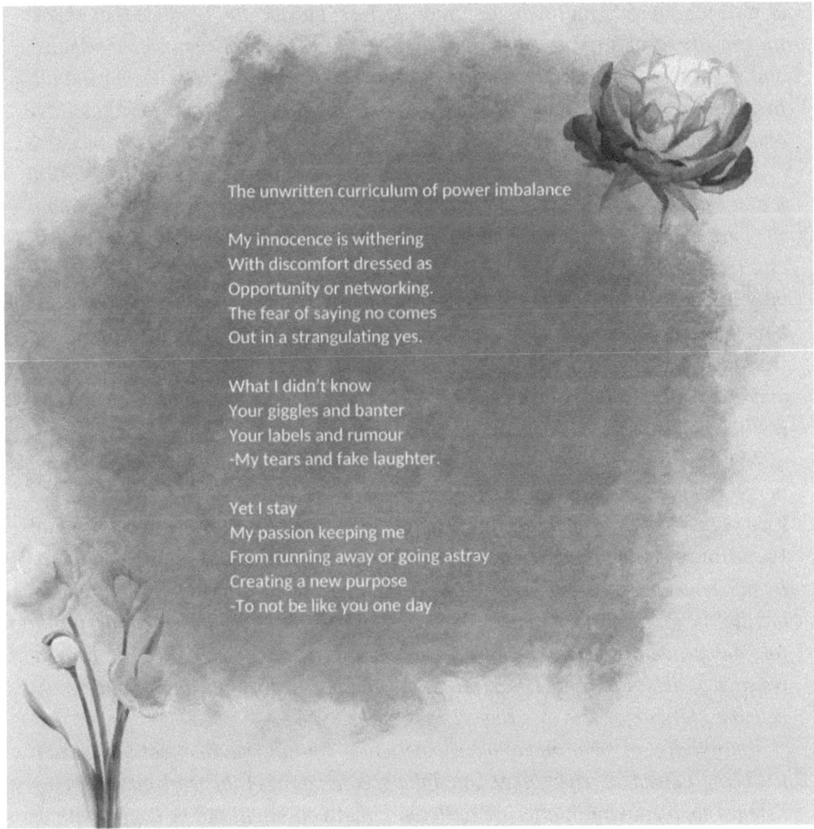

Figure 11.1 The Mental Toll of Doing a PhD (Original Poem)

and status that non-clinical and ex-clinical researchers cannot.[7] We see this tension manifest in the way that MD/PhD programs have been an active topic of discussion, while PhD programs which do not exclusively attract clinicians have not.

What Is It Like to Be a Research Assistant?

Cristina is a research assistant, soon to be a PhD student. Here she reflects on her experience as a doctor working internationally and transitioning to be a researcher in the UK.

It was only when I was offered this position that I realized that I had done this role unofficially before. We participate in data gathering and processing as part of research projects routinely as junior doctors, but we don't realize that this is unofficially what a research assistant does. I embarked on this journey by chance, and it launched me into the world of medical education research like a catapult, in the soft landing of senior support for my curiosity and thirst for knowledge always nurtured by role models.

I'm fortunate to have a remote job, which fits in nicely within my other clinical job in training, and it has also been crucial in maximizing my potential without the burden of my disability. The team that I work with has been very supportive and understanding from the start. Despite being expected to sometimes work out of hours and fill in the gaps of less desired tasks, I've thoroughly enjoyed it and have gained an immeasurable amount of knowledge. The downside of this and working remotely has been that the line between work and life becomes more faded and you need to know how to balance your time and tasks well, otherwise you can easily become overwhelmed.

My first stepping stone was working in a second language, which has been nerve-racking. Despite being an international medical graduate, my team has been patient and non-judgmental throughout. I've never felt the annoyance that I sometimes get in clinical practice when someone doesn't understand me well or I can't remember a word; here I can just be myself and grow. With no previous qualitative research experience, though I had worked within my trade union role independently before, because I work in a very senior-led specialty, being a research assistant at times has felt thrilling and positively daunting. I could never be more grateful for this experience!

I'm mindful of what others have experienced within this role: not being paid, not being named on papers that you did a good amount of the work on, not being listened to, hierarchy interfering with work that you might not be happy with or not have time to do. This is a plea, if you do sign up for an RA role, to reassess these elements as you progress through the role and, if this unpleasantness arises, raise it with your line manager, your team, or just leave. The experience is valuable, but you deserve to be treated fairly, and my experience is a testimony that that is possible.

– Cristina Costache, paediatrics trainee and doctoral student

Cristina's reflection on her experiences of working as a research assistant within medical education is a poem of two halves (Figures 11.2 and 11.3). As with the poems showcasing the highs and lows of living life as a graduate student, the two halves of this poem explore relatively polarizing experiences – of invisibility and bias, but also of mentorship and finding purpose in the field.

There is shockingly little on the role, contributions, and experiences of RAs within medical education. Despite a comprehensive literature search, we could not find anything RAs within medical education

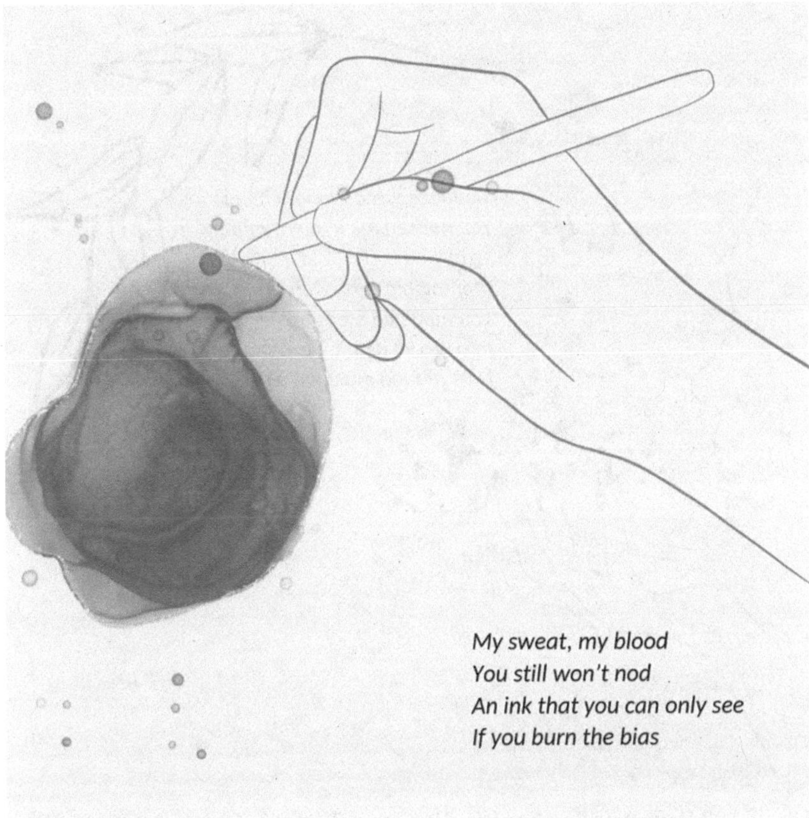

Figure 11.2 Reflections on Work as a Research Assistant (Original Poem)

beyond mentions within academic papers and reports about what project RAs did within data collection and analysis, etc. This is despite the fact that RAs often carry the most significant burden within a research project in terms of participant liaison, data collection, analysis, management, and production of project reports (suggested by the proportion of funding often allocated to RAs' time within grant applications).[8] Without RAs, wider literature notes that much high-impact and grant-funded research would never reach completion, as senior academics are time poor.[8]

Outside of medical education, there are papers which suggest that RAs are "silenced partners" in study knowledge production.[8,9] Hobson, Jones, and Deane[8] comment on the lack of recognition of RAs and their

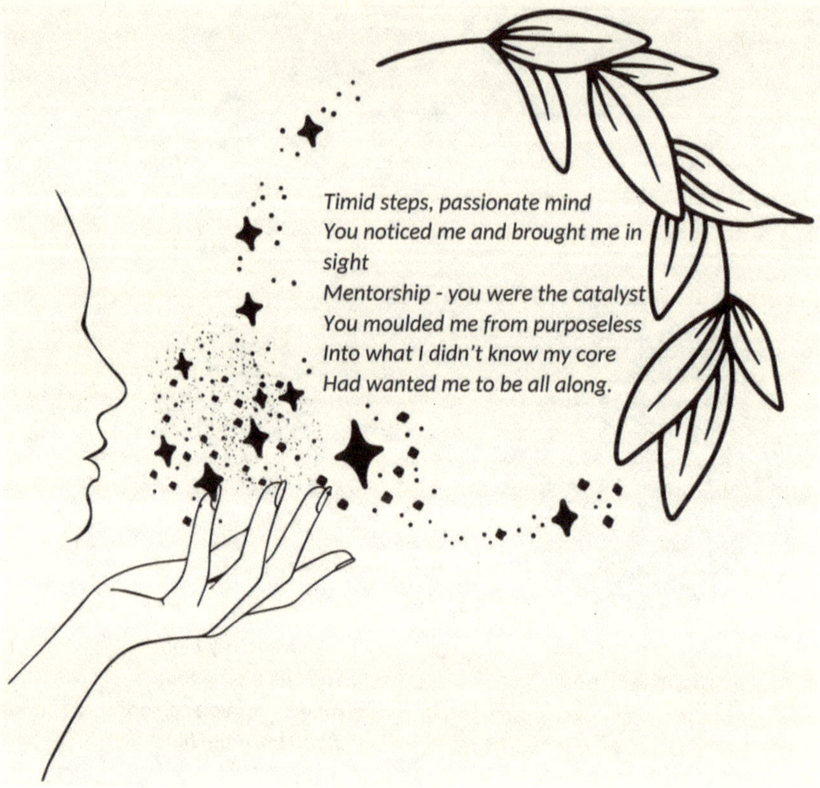

Figure 11.3 Reflections on Contributions as a Research Assistant (Original Poem)

contributions to research projects. This can lead to difficulties defining the role of an RA and comparing the nature and experience within this role across institutions and fields. Where we see the most fruitful and detailed discussion on the topic of RAs outside of medical education, work focuses on undergraduate students' experiences of the RA role[10] which, in nursing, has been suggested translates to an increased interest in clinical academia and evidence-based practice.[11] Though this in-depth exploration and discussion are valuable, they do (perhaps inadvertently) reduce the RA role and its possible impact to an elective experience which any undergraduate student could complete. Given that we also found evidence of belittling of the RA role in wider literature,[12] the hidden message regarding this focus is one that detracts from the advanced skill set and critical impact of the role.

What Is It Like to Be a Supervisor of Graduate Students and Research Assistants?

Gabrielle is an experienced supervisor of graduate students and research assistants; here she reflects on the tensions within the unseen aspects of the role:

I often refer to my graduate students and research assistants as being my family. I want to nurture them and help them fly the nest as fully fledged independent researchers. This group is my pride and joy, and it is such an honour to play a part in their development. I genuinely find supervision to be the most fulfilling part of my job. It is not without its challenges; there is a lot of unseen work that goes into nurturing the individuals and their research. Supervision isn't always easy; not only are you developing each student or assistant as an individual, but there are the team dynamics to nurture too: the unseen unrest, jealousy, angst, the general tensions that can simmer in any group of highly motivated, intelligent individuals. There is no one way to supervise – I have had to learn through trial and error what works for which student. Some need hand-holding, gentle words, and constant reassurance in order to reach their potential; others, direct words, carrots dangled to rev up their innate competitive nature. Learning to maximize the potential of each student while letting them be autonomous, while helping them develop their skills and providing coaching all at once, can be exhausting and requires treading on a very fine line. Not too much that they feel you're taking over, not too little that they feel you don't care. Supervising is a privilege and carries a great deal of responsibility, but it is hard to strike the balance between supporting independent thought, helping to generate ideas, and ultimate owner-ship. A lot of the work a supervisor does, rightly, is not acknowledged as the student flourishes and begins to author papers. Students often forget that their supervisor has been there: we know the struggles first-hand – they are not alone in this. We've experienced the stresses of holding down multiple jobs, of balancing temporary contracts, and taking giant leaps of faith into the academic workforce. A good supervisor should be invisible, cheering on their student in the wings. I want my students to feel that I am there to help lift them up, amplify their voice, and make them feel invincible, not invisible.

– Gabrielle M. Finn, supervisor of graduate students
and research assistants

The poem in Figure 11.4 was co-written by Megan and Gabrielle. Gabrielle is an experienced supervisor of graduate students and research assistants, while Megan is beginning her supervisory journey within medical education. When discussing what it was like to supervise, Gabrielle likened the role to that of a gardener who nurtures and tends

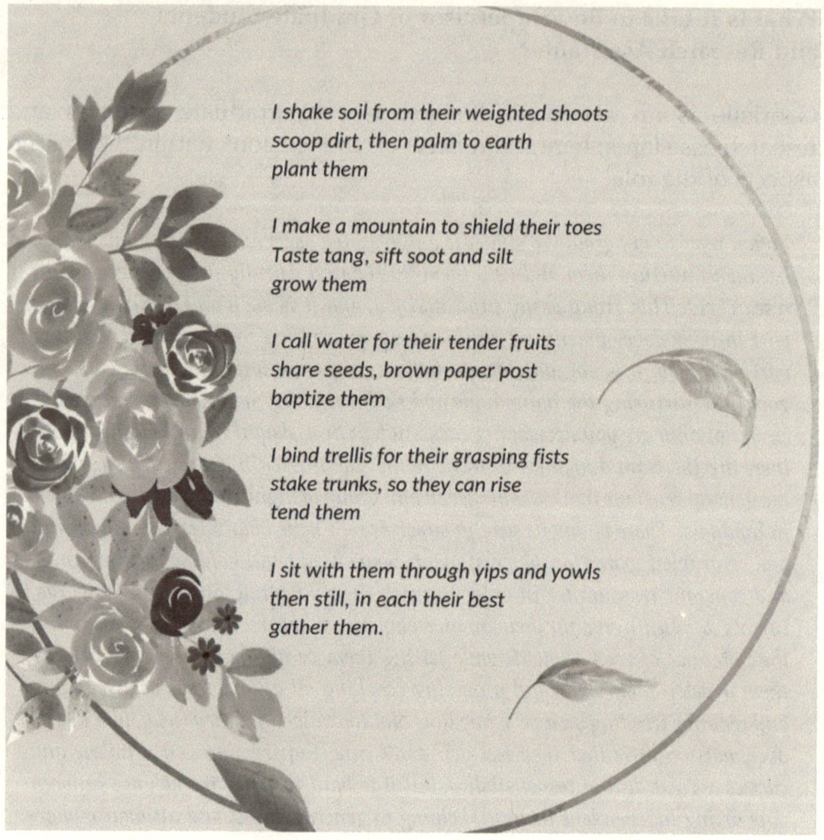

Figure 11.4 Reflections on Supervising Research Trainees (Original Poem)

their garden through all weathers, with great care, while being attentive to creating the most fruitful environment. The poem elaborates on this metaphor.

Though the topic of clinical supervision within medical education is of increasing interest, particularly within educational environments shifting towards competency-based approaches, there has been comparatively little focus on the topic of educational supervision. Similarly, there is a lack of empirical exploration regarding the experience of supervision, and the necessary components of effective and thoughtful graduate student and research assistant supervision. There are, like for graduate students, experience-based commentaries and useful guides offering new supervisors tips on the role and various requirements,[13] but no empirical research on this topic that we could identify within medical education.

In other academic fields, there are some relevant and useful contributions to the literature on the topic of graduate student supervision, including guidance on the need for structured planning,[14] the importance of reflection and feedback,[15] and advice on common issues encountered within supervision (such as academic writing, quality and frequency of meetings, and career advice).[16] Far less common in academic literature is a focus on the supervision of RAs. From the few papers we could identify on this topic, authors note the importance of establishing clear expectations for the RA role, support in developing robust research practices,[17,18] and the value of mentoring within supervisor-RA relationships.[19] Interestingly, and echoing the literature we have synthesized above, the papers we identified on the topic of RA supervision outside of medicine mostly focused on RAs within the context of the RA role as an opportunity for high-performing undergraduate students. Lechuga described the responsibilities of faculty as mentors for graduate students as being that of an ally, ambassador, and master-teacher.[20] While we agree, it is often the other way around – through reverse mentoring for the faculty member, whether we realize it or not.

Silences in the Academic Literature

We have highlighted the silences within the academic literature and gaps when drawing comparisons between the lived experiences of the authors of this chapter and what is formally documented. The experiences of students and their supervisors are largely *empirically* unknown. We do not know how many people work as graduate students and research assistants within medical education, and there is little in the academic literature regarding the role, responsibilities, experiences, and needs of graduate students and research assistants. How these roles function within and contribute to research teams and team dynamics remains unclear. Such silences may stem from the diversity of roles, lack of prestige of an often non-clinical status, and hierarchy within research teams.

Graduate student and RA roles are relatively junior within research teams. This means the status of these roles is likely less (as junior roles often are perceived as lower status within team environments). Further, the roles are associated with relatively low pay and employment insecurity (particularly the RA role, which usually is created to support short-term projects and funding). We could find little on the demographics of the people who become graduate students and RAs (a further silence in the literature), which makes it challenging to draw firm conclusions. Historically, graduate students were only able to study if well supported by family or generational wealth, and issues with funding for graduate studies persist, meaning that access to graduate study opportunities for those from minoritized backgrounds is more challenging. The RA role is a form of casual employment, and so we suspect that minoritized individuals (such as women) are more likely to take on RA employment – wider literature suggests that women are more likely to take on casual employment due to perceived flexibility (although this flexibility rarely manifests in casual roles).[21] Due to bias within higher education and medical education, this increases the likelihood that the RA role will be negatively stereotyped and, largely, ignored.

Why Is This Important?

The effects of medical education research are wide-reaching and, as those of us working in the field know, there is a close connection to clinical practice, both in terms of who is involved in medical education research and outcomes for patient health and social care. Clinicians may be involved in interacting with, or even supervising, research assistants and graduate students working within medical education. As a practical and practice-orientated field, clinical perspectives are valued as a way of enhancing medical education impact. It is, therefore, important for clinicians to appreciate the troubling lack of conversation in regards to RA and graduate student support, and the likely causes of this silence being found in bias and discrimination. Clinicians, as members or leaders of a research team, have active roles in supporting diversity within academic research by appreciating and challenging the intersectional barriers that RAs and graduate students face. Simple acts, such as naming RAs in grant applications where possible or supporting graduate students to participate in grant applications, can improve the visibility of these roles and their impact and provide opportunities for career development. For those with no formal roles in medical education, being mindful of the hidden messages one communicates through interactions with students about the value of medical education research and researchers and ensuring professional conduct with all members of a research team, including the most junior members, are small steps one can immediately take.

It is also important to note that, in clinical practice, clinicians often informally assume the role of an RA. Clinical practice is built on evidence, which, as is widely agreed, is often unfunded, particularly at a local level. The more junior members of a clinical team may be called upon by clinical seniors to develop ideas for local improvement projects, collect and analyse data, present findings, and implement changes. Within the UK, quality improvement is an expectation of a junior doctor's job, for example, that has to be actively evidenced for career progression. When done well, with a supportive clinical senior willing to mentor juniors in research skill development, this can be a mutually beneficial arrangement leading to network-building, skill development, and expanding horizons in terms of areas of research interests and improvement opportunities. We suspect that many clinical seniors have unknowingly assumed the role of RA supervisor in the usual course of their clinical practice. There is a risk that doing so without recognition of the significant responsibility of this role, and the potential challenges and barriers to the trainees' success, may cause harm to all involved and minimize opportunities for enhancing patient care. It is difficult to say no when the medical profession and academia exist in an atmosphere of competition where students feel like they have to stand out,[22] and it can be hard to distinguish where opportunity ends and exploitation starts.

Given these challenges, it is important to consider what we can do to remedy these issues. Challenging this hidden messaging represents an intensely necessary cultural shift which manifests in the discussions that we have and in the people that we surround ourselves with – whether they are people who nourish others or people who take all they can get. As a collective, particularly seniors in positions of organizational power, we must challenge what is inappropriate, make new, inclusive rules, and bend the existing norm. As Shehan Karunatilaka[23] puts it: "You can use your privilege to help others or to exclude them." Carrying this thought, Cristina has written a poem (Figure 11.5) reflecting on the possible damaging effects of the hidden curriculum and power imbalances for those in graduate student or research assistant roles.

Concluding Thoughts

Through our narratives, we have highlighted the important yet often undervalued rules of research assistants and graduate students. Our exploration demonstrated a paucity of literature within our field, leading us to suggest areas for future research. First, there is a need to shift the focus of research exploration to focus on the research team across career stages, their roles, responsibilities, contributions, and experiences. Moreover, defining research assistant and graduate student roles

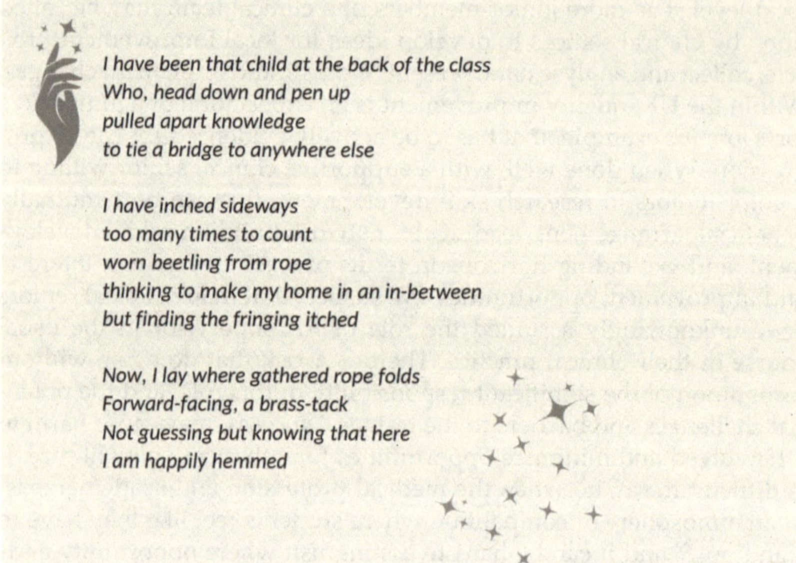

Figure 11.5 The Unwritten Curriculum of Power Imbalance (Original Poem)

explicitly and beginning a conversation regarding standards and career pathways could improve experiences, motivation, productivity, and retention within the field.

The invisibility of the work of these pivotal members of the health professions community potentially underscores the ongoing challenges raised within our narratives and poems, namely those of power imbalances, precarious work conditions, imposter syndrome, and an underappreciation of the nurturing side of supervision.

There is a definite need to collect data on the number of RAs and PhD students within medical education and monitor evolutions in this area. This would be a useful marker of growth, and could provide

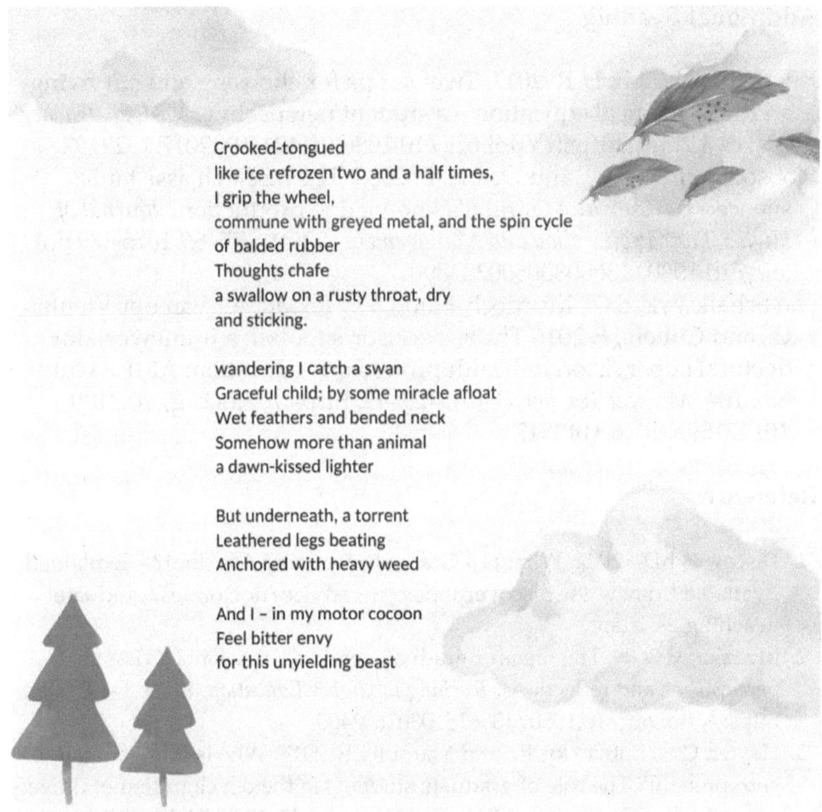

Figure 11.6 Reflections on the Hidden Work of Research (Original Poem)

accurate information on pipeline, bottleneck, and retention. An important aspect that shouldn't be forgotten is equality, diversity, and inclusion, and doing this right: making the distinction between tokenism and meaningful diversity through creating opportunities, valuing lived experience, and supporting diverse potential. The absence of literature is perhaps an indicator of a potential hidden curriculum in this space, namely the tacit message that these roles are not highly valued. Graduate students and research assistants are the foundation upon which our research and teaching are built; without them the landscape of medical education will not flourish.

Additional Reading

Bryan, B., Church, H.R. 2017. Twelve tips for choosing and surviving a PhD in medical education – a student perspective. *Medical Teacher*, 39(11), 1123–7. https://doi.org/10.1080/0142159X.2017.1322192

Hobson, J., Jones, G., and Deane, E. 2005. The research assistant: silenced partner in Australia's knowledge production? *Journal of Higher Education Policy and Management*, 27(3), 357–66. https://doi.org/10.1080/13600800500283890

van Schalkwyk, S.C., Murdoch-Eaton, D., Tekian, A., Van der Vleuten, C., and Cilliers, F. 2016 The supervisor's toolkit: a framework for doctoral supervision in health professions education: AMEE Guide No. 104. *Medical Teacher*, 38(5), 429–42. https://doi.org/10.3109/0142159X.2016.1142517

References

1. DiscoverPhDs. 2022. What Is a Graduate Teaching Assistant? – Explained. Available from: www.discoverphds.com/advice/doctorates/graduate-teaching-assistant.

2. Muzaka, V. 2009. The niche of graduate teaching assistants (GTAs): perceptions and reflections. *Teaching in Higher Education*, 14(1), 1–12. https://doi.org/10.1080/13562510802602400

3. Hayter, C.S., Lubynsky, R., and Maroulis, S. 2017. Who is the academic entrepreneur? The role of graduate students in the development of university spinoffs. *The Journal of Technology Transfer*, 42, 1237–54. https://doi.org/10.1007/s10961-016-9470-y

4. ten Cate, O. 2007. Medical education in the Netherlands. *Medical Teacher*, 29(8), 752–7. https://doi.org/10.1080/01421590701724741

5. Bryan, B., Church, H.R. 2017. Twelve tips for choosing and surviving a PhD in medical education – a student perspective. *Medical Teacher*, 39(11), 1123–7. https://doi.org/10.1080/0142159X.2017.1322192

6. Ciampa, E.J., Hunt, A.A., Arneson, K.O., Mordes, D.A., Oldham, W.M., Woo, K.V., Owens, D.A., Cannon, M.D., and Dermody, T.S. 2011. A workshop on leadership for MD/PhD students. *Medical Education Online*, 16(1). https://doi.org/10.3402/meo.v16i0.7075

7. Church, H., and Brown, M.E.L. 2022. Rise of the Med-Ed-ists: achieving a critical mass of non-practicing clinicians within medical education. *Medical Education*, 56(12). https://doi.org/10.1111/medu.14940

8. Hobson, J., Jones, G., and Deane, E. 2005. The research assistant: silenced partner in Australia's knowledge production? *Journal of Higher Education Policy and Management*, 27(3), 357–66. https://doi.org/10.1080/13600800500283890

9. Nelson, P., and Petrova, M.G. 2022. Research assistants: scientific credit and recognized authorship. *Learned Publishing*, 35(3), 423–7. https://doi.org/10.1002/leap.1467

10. Silva, T.D.N., da Cunha Aguiar, L.C., Leta, J., Santos, D.O., Cardoso, F.S., Cabral, L.M., Rodrigues, C.R., and Castro, H.C. 2004. Role of the undergraduate student research assistant in the new millennium. *Cell Biology Education*, 3(4), 235–40. https://doi.org/10.1187/cbe.04-02-0032

11. Mitchell, K., Rekiere, J., and Grassley, J.S. 2020. The influence of undergraduate research assistant experiences on future nursing roles. *Journal of Professional Nursing*, 36(3), 128–33. https://doi.org/10.1016/j.profnurs.2019.09.006

12. Morison, M., and Moir, J. 1998. The role of computer software in the analysis of qualitative data: efficient clerk, research assistant or Trojan horse? *Journal of Advanced Nursing*, 28(1), 106–16. https://doi.org/10.1046/j.1365-2648.1998.00768.x

13. van Schalkwyk, S.C., Murdoch-Eaton, D., Tekian, A., Van der Vleuten, C., and Cilliers, F. 2016 The supervisor's toolkit: a framework for doctoral supervision in health professions education: AMEE Guide No. 104. *Medical Teacher*, 38(5), 429–42. https://doi.org/10.3109/0142159X.2016.1142517

14. Bitzer, E.M., and Albertyn, R.M. 2011. Alternative approaches to postgraduate supervision: a planning tool to facilitate supervisory processes. *South African Journal of Higher Education*, 25(5), 875–88. https://doi.org/110.4314/SAJHE.V25I5

15. Brew, A., and Peseta, T. 2004. Changing postgraduate supervision practice: a programme to encourage learning through reflection and feedback. *Innovations in Education and teaching International*, 41(1), 5–22. https://doi.org/10.1080/1470329032000172685

16. Caldwell, P.H., Oldmeadow, W., and Jones, C.A. 2012. Supervisory needs of research doctoral students in a university teaching hospital setting. *Journal of Paediatrics and Child Health*, 48(10), 907–12. https://doi.org/10.1111/j.1440-1754.2012.02522.x

17. Maher, M.A., Gilmore, J.A., Feldon, D.F., and Davis, T.E. 2013. Cognitive apprenticeship and the supervision of science and engineering research assistants. *Journal of Research Practice*, 9(2), M5. Accessible from: http://jrp.icaap.org/index.php/jrp/article/view/354/311

18. Gift, A.G., Creasia, J., and Parker, B. 1991. Utilizing research assistants and maintaining research integrity. *Research in Nursing & Health*, 14(3), 229–33. https://doi.org/10.1002/nur.4770140310

19. Whiteside, U., Pantelone, D.W., Hunter-Reel, D., Eland, J., Kleiber, B., and Larimer, M. 2007. Initial suggestions for supervising and mentoring undergraduate research assistants at large research universities. *International Journal of Teaching & Learning in Higher Education*, 19(3), 325–30.

20. Lechuga, V.M. 2011. Faculty-graduate student mentoring relationships: mentors' perceived roles and responsibilities. *Higher Education*, 62:757–71. https://doi.org/10.1007/s10734-011-9416-0
21. Pocock, B.A., Prosser, R.W., and Bridge, K.J. 2004. Only a casual ... how casual work affects employees, households and communities in Australia. University of Adelaide.
22. Lempp, H., and Seale, C. 2004. The hidden curriculum in undergraduate medical education: qualitative study of medical students' perceptions of teaching. *BMJ*, 329(7469), 770–3. https://doi.org/10.1136/bmj.329.7469.770
23. Karunatilaka, S. 2022. *The Seven Moons of Maali Almeida*. Sort of Books.

12 The Invisible Work of Librarians in Health Professions Education

LOUISE ALLEN, PALLAVI PRATHIVADI,
AND LINDSEY SIKORA

I often joke how librarians are the hairstylists of the academic world – where we are often used as a sounding board for issues arising from students, faculty, and administrators – yet the implications are serious in nature. We not only play a pivotal role in educating young physicians from the start of their medical career, but we are also in a unique position to listen to everyone in the medical education community without bias. We are able to listen to all sides yet play a neutral role in bringing together community members to ensure that everyone is being listened to, while ensuring that the quality of education and research is being properly obtained. We hear perspectives from those who may not feel comfortable or safe sharing their views with others, allowing us to broach topics in a neutral way to move ideas forward.

– Lindsey Sikora, medical librarian, Head of Research Support
(Health Sciences, Medicine, STEM)

For many of us, our first experience with librarians is as children, either at school or at a library within the community. There, librarians give us access to a range of resources we might not be able to access otherwise – books, music, and computers with the Internet, just to name a few. As we progress through school, librarians can help us find resources to complete assignments. Often when we think of librarians, we think of a friendly face that can expand our world beyond what we currently understand. This rings true within medical education and healthcare, as librarians are not only able to show students, faculty, and patients where to find information, but they also show them *how* to find information, empowering them to seek out evidence-based medicine.

In this chapter, we will explore the invisible work of librarians in all phases of medical education. We explore the vast range of roles that librarians have in medical education, and the contributions they make to educating future and current physicians. Librarians go far beyond providing access to resources and assisting students and clinicians with searching for answers to their questions. They help medical students develop into competent clinicians equipped with the variety of skills they need to effectively practise evidence-based medicine; they help clinicians to continue to upskill and can assist with improving decision-making; and they ultimately contribute to improving patient care. The role of medical librarians is so integral to the training, development, and evidence-based practice of physicians that this chapter has been intentionally written in a collaborative multi-lens perspective by a medical librarian, a medical education academic, and a practising academic physician. Together, we argue that while librarians are integral to medical education, they are underutilized and under-recognized, with much of their work being invisible. We propose why this might be the case and offer some suggestions for how this may be rectified.

Librarians in Medical Education: A Collaborative Academic Perspective

The librarian profession is an ancient one, being traced back to hundreds of years BC.[1] Consequently, considerable shifts in librarians' roles have occurred. Traditionally, librarians were confined to the library, their roles focusing on maintaining, cataloguing, and distributing knowledge from physical resources.[2] Those seeking access to the library's resources were required to visit the library and work with a librarian. Thus, the library provided a space for knowledge sharing, development, and community. However, with a range of advances in computerized bibliographic systems beginning in the 1960s, the development of the Internet in the 1980s, and the emergence of online databases and electronic journals, the ability for individuals to search and access libraries' resources without the aid of a librarian has grown.[2,3] This necessitated the expansion of the library and librarians into the virtual space, with education and support occurring in both the physical library and online. It also led to the shift of librarians being solely located in libraries to librarians working within context, such as being embedded and located in a medical school. Librarians' roles have expanded accordingly to include effectively searching, appraising, and synthesizing large volumes of evidence, as well as teaching these crucial skills to others while providing resources that assist with these skills.

In medicine, the evolution of librarians' roles has continued. A growing focus on evidence-based medicine (EBM) globally is evidenced by the introductions of competencies such as the practice-based learning and improvement competency by the Accreditation Council for

Table 12.1 Librarian assistance

Medical Students[31]

- Identifying and formulating important clinical and research questions for investigation.
- Identifying the relevance of their project to medicine and healthcare.
- Learning the appropriate approaches to addressing their question based on methodological standards to the relevant fields of study.
- Learning how to formulate a clinical or research question and to search for and critically appraise the available evidence.
- Designing, conducting, and interpreting the results of their projects based on the question and methodological approaches.
- Effectively communicating the results in oral and written form.
- Ensuring ethics and professionalism are kept throughout their project.

Trainees, Junior Doctors and Physicians[12,32–34]

- Access to medical literature: Helping doctors find and access medical literature, including peer-reviewed articles, textbooks, and other resources that can help them learn about new treatments, procedures, and research in their field.
- Research assistance: Assisting doctors with their research needs, such as helping them conduct literature searches, access databases, and find reliable sources of information.
- Evidence-based practice: Helping doctors to stay up to date and to understand the importance of evidence-based practice and assist them in finding, appraising, synthesizing, and using the best available evidence to inform their clinical decisions.
- Information literacy: Teaching doctors how to evaluate sources of information and distinguish between reliable and unreliable information, helping them develop critical thinking and information literacy skills.

Graduate Medical Education in the USA,[4,5] the Royal College of Physicians and Surgeons of Canada CanMEDS scholar competency,[6] and the Australian Medical Council's Graduate Outcome Statements Science and Scholarship domain.[7] They all specifically refer to the ability to appraise, interpret, and apply evidence in practice. As librarians possess a range of skills to assist with these competencies, the role of librarians in medical education has now evolved to the point where they are involved at all levels of medical education: medical school (undergraduate or postgraduate),[8–11] graduate medical education,[12–14] and continuing education (CE).[15–18] Furthermore, across all levels of medical education, librarians' roles go beyond managing and distributing information to involvement in teaching and education, scholarship and research, and clinical care. The following paragraphs provide an overview of each of these roles, and Table 12.1 provides a summary of the ways in which librarians assist medical students, trainees, junior doctors, and physicians.

Librarians assume a range of roles in teaching and education that differ across institutions.[19,20] These roles range from librarians based solely within the library, to librarians delivering guest lectures, to highly integrated librarians who are part of course or curriculum committees and are heavily involved in the design, delivery, assessment, and evaluation of teaching and education, and everything in between.[20] Beyond medical school and training programs, librarians are increasingly being involved in CE for physicians. For example, they are members of continuing medical education committees where they can assist with needs assessments and identifying practice gaps to assist with the construction of relevant CE.[16,17]

Scholarship and research roles include lending their expertise to medical students, trainees, or junior doctors, and physicians with respect to searching the literature – particularly in review methodology, research question formulation, development, and implementation of search strategies, conducting and documenting searches, and writing the search methods.[21,22] Evidence shows that librarians' involvement as a co-author or team member in conducting reviews improves the quality of reviews.[23,24]

In terms of clinical care, clinical librarians work alongside medical students, trainees or junior doctors, and physicians to "provide quality assured information to health professionals at the point of need to support clinical decision-making."[25 (p. 17)] This can involve attending morning report or ward rounds and utilizing their searching, appraisal, and knowledge-synthesis skills to answer questions in the moment. Clinical librarians provide a number of benefits to clinical care, including improved clinical decision-making and patient care, reduced length of stay, savings in terms of both time and money, reducing adverse events, and enhancing evidence-based practice.[16,26–30]

But despite such diverse roles in medical education, librarians are under-recognized and underutilized.[12,35,36] A survey of library instruction in medical education in the USA and Canada showed that while 90 per cent (n=73) of respondents indicated they offered instruction that is embedded in the curriculum in at least one academic year, only 4 per cent offered instruction that is embedded in the curriculum in all four years of medical school.[35] While a survey of paediatric residency program directors showed that 81 per cent (n=91) of programs engage medical librarians, the most common role (74 per cent) was assisting with scholarly or research projects. Only 17 per cent of programs had librarians engaged in teaching EBM regularly, and only 8 per cent of programs had medical librarians involved in curriculum development.[12] This is a problem for multiple reasons: i) it demonstrates that librarians aren't being used to their full potential in medical education; ii) it devalues the expertise and unique skills librarians have beyond assisting with research such as contributing to EBM competencies; iii) it shows others who may not have the same expertise in EBM are being engaged in this work rather than librarians; and iv) it contributes to librarians' work being invisible as librarians aren't given the opportunity to utilize these skills, and learners and other educators may therefore not see the role or value librarians provide.

To illustrate the invisible work of librarians, we highlight perspectives of two individuals actively working in medical education: Pallavi Prathivadi, an academic primary care physician, who provides a clinical perspective on the importance of librarians; and Lindsey Sikora, Head of Research Support (Health Sciences, Medicine, STEM), who highlights the responsibilities and challenges that librarians experience throughout medical education.

Librarians in Medical Education: A Physician's Perspective

I do not recall a meaningful interaction with a medical librarian through five years of medical school, an honours research year, four years of hospital jobs as a junior doctor, or the three years of specialist general practice training and fellowship. It was 12 years after starting medical school, as a first year PhD candidate, that I was first encouraged by a non-medical supervisor to contact the university medical librarian after submitting an embarrassingly written study protocol with a literature review largely conducted using Google (the regular version; I only learned about Google Scholar after that first meeting with the librarian)."
– Pallavi Prathivadi, academic primary care physician

Academic medicine and research are almost universally core aspects of medical training and practice. Clinical practice requires skills in knowledge synthesis and decision-making which are guided by protocol-driven procedures, intuitive reasoning, and application of best-practice evidence. In early university or campus-based years, medical students require skills in searching, knowledge access, and research methods and theory. Librarians are experts in these skill sets and are well placed to form part of the team that assists students and doctors to develop these professional competencies. However, librarians are commonly not considered or given formal opportunities to train or educate medical learners. Instead, pervasive attitudes in the medical communities imply that these research skills can be satisfactorily delivered by "others," including senior doctors, collegial academics, and peers without formal research training. Unfortunately, this perpetuates the standard that "we (physicians) don't know what we don't know."

The skills that we are not usually formally taught are certainly needed in daily clinical practice and modern patient care, according to patients, administrative staff, nursing staff, hospital leadership, families, and even the general public.[37] Similarly, clinical or hospital-based students may require guidance in patient-centred clinical research. They are also frequently given opportunities to present patient cases during ward rounds, multidisciplinary discussions, and morbidity and mortality meetings. This usually involves a short synopsis of the key clinical aspects of the patient's case followed by an in-depth discussion of pathophysiology or evidence-based treatment recommendations. As a student, these are typically stressful and intimidating activities; presenting clinical recommendations to specialists with decades of experience instils a great fear of being incorrect and undermined in front of senior (and future) medical colleagues. Hospital librarians could have key roles in supporting students in searching the literature and knowledge synthesis to prepare up-to-date and relevant content for a reliable and informative clinical presentation. Indeed, with the help of a librarian, ward rounds and grand rounds could be even more educationally rich for the learners and for the attendings.

When it comes to research, many Western specialist medical training programs have mandatory research terms or projects that necessitate an expected level of research expertise. Clinician-researcher careers like mine which combine clinical practice and research increase intellectual stimulation, improve our evidence-based practice, and provide more opportunities to make scientific discoveries to advance patient care and medicine.[38] Despite this, formal training or higher research degrees such as PhDs are held by less than 10 per cent of physicians.[39] Increasing efforts to engage medical doctors in research include targeted clinician-researcher funding schemes, opportunities for dual training in research and clinical practice, and MD-PhD degree programs.[39]

Earlier exposure to research can prepare and encourage pursuit of academic medical careers.[40] However, inclusion of specific research skill development in medical curricula is often far less vigorous compared to non-medical science programs. Less than one-fifth of research projects in medical school provide opportunity for skill development in all four research areas; research methods, information gathering, critical analysis and review, and data processing.[41] In my own undergraduate medical degree, the opportunity for comprehensive research skills development was offered as a one-year sabbatical from medical school to undertake an entire three-year honours research degree in a short

10 months. Although this was a pathway I selected (and which influenced my later academic career), competing clinical interests, lack of research expertise of teachers/trainers, pressure to graduate and advance medical careers, and wide scope of curriculum material in generalist medical degrees were common barriers to both my peers and medical students internationally in engaging with research. Access to librarians with expertise in medical literature and health curricula may help address many such barriers and support medical schools to develop reputed and vigorous research training and clinician-scientist degree programs.

Productive and collegial relationships between experienced medical librarians and medical students can also support capacity-building and knowledge translation. Despite increasing pushback from physician and surgical specialists,[42,43] international medical culture still persists in using the "see one, do one, teach one" approach whereby a learner firstly observes a skill being performed by another, then later attempts the skill themselves, and then completes the skill cycle by teaching the skill to a (more) novice learner.[44] This learning approach is widespread across many clinical and non-clinical skills, including emergency procedures, surgical procedures, and medical ethics.[42,45,46] Medical students also commonly engage in group study to share knowledge through social learning and peer influence.[47] This includes formal university tutorials, student-organized study groups, and also informal enjoyment-based socialization with peers and friends where knowledge is still exchanged. Students can therefore disseminate instruction and knowledge gained from interactions with librarians in both "see one, do one, teach one" or in group skill-sharing methods. In turn, this may improve research skills in a larger population of students, increase the likelihood of engaging in academic roles or higher research degrees, and improve the visibility of the role and value of librarians. Increasing positive perceptions of librarians by medical students and doctors should then help increase recognition and value of these key members of medical academic teams and improve librarian authorship rates and funding.[48] Doctors currently providing education and training to medical learners may not have collaborated with librarians during their own medical training and therefore fail to recognize the benefits and opportunities this offers. My own professional pathway as a dual trained clinician-scientist has led me to recognize how librarians could be really valuable assets to medical education:

Reflecting on my own experiences, I can now easily outline the multitude of opportunities for medical students to engage with medical librarians, but I certainly did not at the time. It may be an example of "you don't know what you don't know." Only after working closely with medical librarians for four years of my PhD to prepare study methodology, register systematic review protocols, submit grant applications, undertake reviews with international universities, source grey literature and unpublished data, and more do I see the opportunities I missed in earlier years. As a generalist physician and primary care academic, I appreciate the multidisciplinary influence and approach that provides best patient care and also recognize that transdisciplinary insights (from relevant topics in law, engineering, finance, literature, economics, and more) can be groundbreaking to many medical advances. Librarians, certainly, should be considered as valuable interdisciplinary peers for doctors, but they also bring wide transdisciplinary knowledge themselves. The missed opportunities for medical students to receive guidance and instruction from librarians disadvantages us and our careers, and we have a great deal to learn from non-medical colleagues more generally.

– Pallavi Prathivadi

Librarians in Medical Education: A Librarian's Perspective

One of the most interesting aspects of being a medical librarian is the various roles we play in medical education. When well integrated, librarians are involved in many aspects of medical education, including teaching and education (curriculum design and delivery), scholarship and research, and clinical care.

I think it's important to mention that while many librarians do work in academic institutions, there are others that work outside of academia. There are many librarians that work in hospital settings and specialized libraries that also actively teach, collaborate, and participate in the scholarship of medical students, residents, and physicians."

– Lindsey Sikora

The sheer number of ways that librarians do make (and could make more) meaningful contributions to medical education is hard to summarize because the expertise of handling the ever-growing knowledge base is one that is relevant across all aspects of the field. Librarians can play an important role in curriculum design in medical schools by providing expertise in information management, teaching, and assessment. Through collaboration with faculty, librarians can identify gaps in the curriculum where information literacy and research skills may be lacking. They can provide suggestions for integrating information literacy skills into existing courses or help design new courses that focus on information management and evidence-based practice. Medical librarians can also help develop learning objectives that focus on information literacy and research skills, ensuring that the curriculum meets the needs of medical students and prepares them for their future roles as physicians. Through instructional support to faculty, librarians can teach information literacy and research skills, including developing instructional materials, leading workshops, and providing one-on-one consultations with students. They can also help assess student learning by developing and administering assessments that measure information literacy and research skills, as well as providing feedback to faculty on how to improve these skills in future courses. Lastly, librarians can help ensure that the curriculum stays current by staying up to date with emerging trends in information management and research methods. They can provide suggestions for new technologies or resources that could be incorporated into the curriculum to improve student learning. Through their involvement, librarians can help ensure that medical students are well prepared for their future roles as physicians. In some contexts, medical educators collaborate with librarians to harness these advantages; however, unfortunately, many potential collaborations with librarians are never realized. The skills and support that librarians could offer are often, regrettably, untapped.

As medical students move forward in their career, graduating from medical school to become trainees and junior doctors, their education continues often with an increased focus on scholarship and research as well as direct clinical care. Librarians build upon the skills that medical students have learned as they continue on their path to become physicians. Often, trainees and junior doctors work in hospitals other than where they went to medical school and have to navigate their new institution's library system; librarians can assist with this transition. While there has been an increased provision of instruction by librarians in medical schools,[35] many librarians are isolated from departments within the medical school, limiting their ability to collaborate with faculty and students on research projects or other initiatives.

Another reason that librarians may be underutilized is the lack of institutional support. This can include insufficient funding for resources, inadequate staffing, and lack of support for professional development opportunities. Lastly, faculty and students may not be aware of the expertise that medical librarians bring to the table. This can result in missed opportunities for collaboration and support, as well as a failure to recognize the value that librarians can add to the medical school community.[49,50] Despite the myriad of roles and crucial contribution of librarians to the development of competent physicians, the lack of acknowledgment of the work of librarians in medical education and practice is a real problem:

I think that one of the largest unacknowledged aspects of being a librarian working in medical education is invisible labour. Invisible labour is necessary work that contributes to a project but often goes unrecognized and unpaid. Librarians often contribute a great deal of time, resources, and energy into preparing teaching materials, handouts, and resources for workshops that are often one-shot sessions. Each individual session needs to be tailored to the course, with specific examples required for that specific session. Finding examples is time consuming as the librarian wants to ensure they are clearly communicating all the information to the participants.

Another example of invisible labour is the searching that goes into a knowledge-synthesis project such as a systematic review or a scoping review. Often, researchers don't understand that librarians spend HOURS creating and revising the search for **one** *database before translating it into other databases, which has a different set of controlled vocabulary and searching components. We ensure that the search is also peer reviewed before we translate it into another database to ensure the quality of search is top notch, as we know that the quality of the review depends on it. But frequently, the intellectual contribution of search development goes without recognition, as the librarian is not granted authorship, which is one of the critical ways to demonstrate value and make a librarian's work visible. Similarly, the search process is devalued by the choice of the language used to describe the search, as pointed out in a great article written by Amanda Ross-White entitled "Search is a verb: Systematic review searching as invisible labor."[51] Advocating for co-authorship and named acknowledgment in these reviews is important beyond the personal impact of a librarian's career. By establishing the importance of this invisible labour, librarians demonstrate the value to other researchers who may lack the awareness of the intellectual work involved in developing the research question and translating it into a comprehensive search. Furthermore, many researchers, as well as library and university administrators, lack familiarity with the work involved in searching, often not providing recognition for this work, which has value and needs to be appropriately given credit. This lack of familiarity can lead to limitations in providing services to students and faculty, especially if there are not enough resources (time, persons) allocated to support these services.*

– Lindsey Sikora

Concluding Thoughts

With our continued and increasing focus on evidence-based medicine and the benefits that librarians provide in terms of medical student, trainee and junior doctor, and physician development, as well as the delivery of safe, effective healthcare, it is clear that librarians should be an essential part of the medical education team. Their involvement is foundational to medical education, as their expertise has demonstrated in this chapter. However, they often do not get the opportunity to be integrated members of medical education teams. And there is room for more consistent involvement of librarians across the medical education spectrum, providing contributions beyond just scholarship and research. This lack of opportunity for librarians disadvantages medical students, junior doctors, and physicians, and therefore ultimately patient care. Steps should be taken to increase the utilization and recognition of librarians in medical education, including more investment from administrators in libraries, universities, and hospitals to support the increased integration of librarians into education and clinical practice; recognizing librarians' contributions to knowledge syntheses, grant proposals, and other scholarship with authorship; and encouraging individual librarians to promote their expertise, thus building their recognition of value to become further integrated in medical education.

Additional Reading

Bullers, K., Howard, A.M., Hanson, A., Kearns, W.D., Orriola, J.J., Polo, R.L., and Sakmar, K.A. 2018. It takes longer than you think: librarian time spent on systematic review tasks. *Journal of the Medical Library Association*, 106(2), 198–207. https://doi.org/10.5195/jmla .2018.323

Divall, P., James C., Heaton, M., and Brettle, A. 2022. UK survey demonstrates a wide range of impacts attributable to clinical librarian services. *Health Information and Libraries Journal*, 39(2), 116–31. https://doi.org/10.1111/hir.12389

Nevius, A.M., Ettien, A.L., Link, A.P., and Sobel, L.Y. 2018. Library instruction in medical education: a survey of current practices in the United States and Canada. *Journal of the Medical Library Association*, 106(1), 98–107. https://doi.org/10.5195/jmla.2018.374

Ross-White, A. 2021. Search is a verb: systematic review searching as invisible labor. *Journal of the Medical Library Association*, 109(3), 505–6. https://doi.org/10.5195/jmla.2021.1226

Wu, L. and Mi, M. 2013. Sustaining librarian vitality: embedded librarianship model for health sciences libraries. *Medical Reference Services Quarterly*, 32(3), 257–65. https://doi.org/10.1080/02763869.2013 .806860

References

1. Winger, H.W. 1961. Aspects of librarianship: a trace work of history. *The Library Quarterly*, 31(4), 321–35. https://doi.org/10.1086/618925

2. Cooper, I.D., and Crum, J.A. 2013. New activities and changing roles of health sciences librarians: a systematic review, 1990–2012. *Journal of the Medical Library Association*, 101(4), 268–77. https://doi.org/10.3163/1536-5050.101.4.008

3. McClure, L.W. 2013. When the librarian was the search engine: introduction to the special issue on new roles for health sciences librarians. *Journal of the Medical Library Association*, 101(4), 257–61. https://doi.org/10.3163/1536-5050.101.4.006

4. Accreditation Council for Graduate Medical Education. 2023. *ACGME Common Program Requirements (Residency)*. Accessed January 23, 2023. Available from: www.acgme.org/globalassets/pfassets/programrequirements/cprresidency_2022v3.pdf

5. Accreditation Council for Graduate Medical Education. 2023. *ACGME Common Program Requirements (Fellowship)*. Accessed January 23, 2023. Available from: https://www.acgme.org/globalassets/pfassets/programrequirements/2025-reformatted-requirements/cprfellowship_2025_reformatted.pdf

6. Frank, J.R., Snell, L., Sherbino, J., eds. 2015. *CanMEDS 2015 Physician Competency Framework*. Royal College of Physicians and Surgeons of Canada.

7. Australian Medical Council. 2023. *Standards for Assessment and Accreditation of Primary Medical Programs*. Australian Medical Council Limited. Accessed March 1, 2023. Available from: www.amc.org.au/wp-content/uploads/2019/10/Standards-for-Assessment-and-Accreditation-of-Primary-Medical-Programs-by-the-Australian-Medical-Council-2012.pdf

8. Akers, K.G., Hu, E., Rehman, N., Yun, H.J., Hoofman, J., Monconduit, R., and Mendez, J. 2022. Building first-year medical students' skills in finding, evaluating, and visualizing health Information through a "debunking medical myths" curricular module. *Medical Science Educator*, 32(2), 309–13. https://doi.org/10.1007/s40670-022-01541-w

9. Gaines, J.K., Blake, L., Kouame, G., Davies, K.J., Ballance, D., Thomas Gaddy, V., Gallman, E., Russell, M., and Wood, E. 2018. Partnering to analyze selection of resources by medical students for case-based small group learning: a collaboration between librarians and medical educators. *Medical Reference Services Quarterly*, 37(3), 249–65. https://doi.org/10.1080/02763869.2018.1477709

10. Maggio, L.A., Durieux, N., and Tannery, N.H. 2015. Librarians in evidence-based medicine curricula: a qualitative study of librarian roles, training, and desires for future development. *Medical Reference Services Quarterly*, 34(4), 428–40. https://doi.org/10.1080/02763869.2015.1082375

11. Premji, Z., Fuller, K., and Raworth R. 2020. A cross-sectional survey on academic librarian involvement in evidence-based medicine instruction within undergraduate medical education programs in Canada. *Journal of*

the Canadian Health Libraries Association, 41(3), 104–25. https://doi.org
/10.29173/jchla29458

12. Boykan, R., and Jacobson, R.M. 2017. The role of librarians in teaching
    evidence-based medicine to pediatric residents: a survey of pediatric resi-
    dency program directors. *Journal of the Medical Library Association*, 105(4),
    355–60. https://doi.org/10.5195/jmla.2017.178

13. Herrmann, L.E., Winer, J.C., Kern, J., Keller, S., and Pavuluri, P. 2017.
    Integrating a clinical librarian to increase trainee application of evidence-
    based medicine on patient family-centered rounds. *Academic Pediatrics*,
    17(3), 339–41. https://doi.org/10.1016/j.acap.2016.11.005

14. Lovasik, B.P., Rutledge, H., Lawson, E., Maithel, S.K., and Delman. K.A.
    2020. Development of a surgical evidence blog at morbidity and mortality
    conferences: integrating clinical librarians to enhance resident education.
    Journal of Surgical Education, 77(5), 1069–75. https://doi.org/10.1016
    /j.jsurg.2020.03.024

15. Babineau, J., Zhao, J., Dubin, R., Taenzer, P., Flannery, J.F., and Furlan, A.D.
    2018. The embedded librarian in a telehealth continuing medical educa-
    tion program. *Journal of Hospital Librarianship*, 18(1), 1–14. https://doi.org
    /10.1080/15323269.2018.1400346

16. Bartkowiak, B.A., Safford, L.A., and Stratman, E.J. 2014. Assessing the
    impact of a medical librarian on identification of valid and actionable
    practice gaps for a continuing medical education committee. *Journal of
    Continuing Education in the Health Professions*, 34(3), 186–94. https://doi.org
    /10.1002/chp.21244

17. Gerber, A.L. 2017. The librarian's contribution to continuing medical edu-
    cation. *Medical Reference Services Quarterly*, 36(4), 408–14. https://doi.org
    /10.1080/02763869.2017.1369291

18. Price, C., Kudchadkar, S.R., Basyal, P.S., Nelliot, A., Smith, M., Friedman,
    M., and Needham, D.M. 2020. Librarian integration into health care
    conferences: a case report. *Journal of the Medical Library Association*, 108(2),
    278–85. https://doi.org/10.5195/jmla.2020.803

19. Linton, A.M. 2016. Emerging roles for librarians in the medical school cur-
    riculum and the impact on professional identity. *Medical Reference Services
    Quarterly*, 35(4), 414–33. https://doi.org/10.1080/02763869.2016.1220758

20. Wu, L., and Mi, M. 2013. Sustaining librarian vitality: embedded librarian-
    ship model for health sciences libraries. *Medical Reference Services Quar-
    terly*, 32(3), 257–65. https://doi.org/10.1080/02763869.2013.806860

21. Bullers, K., Howard, A.M., Hanson, A., Kearns, W.D., Orriola, J.J., Polo,
    R.L., and Sakmar, K.A. 2018. It takes longer than you think: librarian time
    spent on systematic review tasks. *Journal of the Medical Library Association*,
    106(2), 198–207. https://doi.org/10.5195/jmla.2018.323

22. Dudden, R.F., and Protzko, S.L. 2011. The systematic review team: contributions of the health sciences librarian. *Medical Reference Services Quarterly*, 30(3), 301–15. https://doi.org/10.1080/02763869.2011.590425

23. Meert, D., Torabi, N., and Costella, J. 2016. Impact of librarians on reporting of the literature searching component of pediatric systematic reviews. *Journal of the Medical Library Association*, 104(4), 267–77. https://doi.org/10.3163/1536-5050.104.4.004

24. Rethlefsen, M.L., Farrell, A.M., Osterhaus Trzasko, L.C., and Brigham, T.J. 2015. Librarian co-authors correlated with higher quality reported search strategies in general internal medicine systematic reviews. *Journal of Clinical Epidemiology*, 68(6), 617–26. https://doi.org/10.1016/j.jclinepi.2014.11.025

25. Hill, P. 2008. *Report of a National Review of NHS Funded Library Information Services in England: From Knowledge to Health in the 21st Century*. Available from: https://www.researchgate.net/publication/265266144

26. Banks, D.E., Runhua, S.H.I., Timm, D.F., Christopher, K.A., Duggar, D.C., Comegys, M., and McLarty, J. 2007. Decreased hospital length of stay associated with presentation of cases at morning report with librarian support. *Journal of the Medical Library Association*, 95(4), 381–7. https://doi.org/10.3163/1536-5050.95.4.381

27. Brettle, A., Maden, M., Payne, C. 2016. The impact of clinical librarian services on patients and health care organisations. *Health Information and Libraries Journal*, 33(2), 100–120. https://doi.org/10.1111/hir.12136

28. Brettle, A., Maden-Jenkins, M., Anderson, L., McNally, R., Pratchett, T., Tancock, J., Thornton, D., and Webb, A. 2011. Evaluating clinical librarian services: a systematic review. *Health Information and Libraries Journal* , 28(1), 3–22. https://doi.org/10.1111/j.1471-1842.2010.00925.x

29. Divall, P., James C., Heaton, M., and Brettle, A. 2022. UK survey demonstrates a wide range of impacts attributable to clinical librarian services. *Health Information and Libraries Journal*, 39(2), 116–31. https://doi.org/10.1111/hir.12389

30. Marshall, J.G., Sollenberger, J., Easterby-Gannett, S., Morgan, L.K., Klem, M.L., Cavanaugh, S.K., Oliver, K.B., Thompson, C.A., Romanosky, N., and Hunter, S. 2013. The value of library and information services in patient care: results of a multisite study. *Journal of the Medical Library Association*, 101(1), 38–46. https://doi.org/10.3163/1536-5050.101.1.007

31. Zeigen, L., and Hamilton, A. 2021. Evolving librarian engagement in undergraduate medical education student research and scholarship. *Medical Reference Services Quarterly*, 40(3), 337–46. https://doi.org/10.1080/02763869.2021.1945871

32. Howlett, A. 2018. Medical librarians may be underutilised in EBM training within pediatric resident programs. *Evidence Based Library and information Practice*, 13(4), 105–7. https://doi.org/10.18438/eblip29418

33. Kovach, F.E., Brenham, C., Kelley, R.S., Gordon, C.P., and Poole, C. 2013. Family physicians inquiries network (FPIN): librarians connecting with faculty, residents, and medical students to advance evidence-based practice through scholarly publishing. *Journal of Hospital Librarianship*, 13(1), 59–65. https://doi.org/10.1080/15323269.2013.743366

34. Orchanian-Cheff, A., and Kaasa, B. 2022. How to answer clinical questions at the point of care: clinical librarian intervention for family medicine residents. *Canadian Family Physician*, 68(5), e146–50. https://doi.org/10.46747/cfp.6805e146

35. Nevius, A.M., Ettien, A.L., Link, A.P., and Sobel, L.Y. 2018. Library instruction in medical education: a survey of current practices in the United States and Canada. *Journal of the Medical Library Association*, 106(1), 98–107. https://doi.org/10.5195/jmla.2018.374

36. Nicholson, J., Spak, J.M., Kovar-Gough, I., Lorbeer, E.R., and Adams, N.E. 2019. Entrustable professional activity 7: opportunities to collaborate on evidence-based medicine teaching and assessment of medical students. *BMC Medical Education*, 19(1), 330. https://doi.org/10.1186/s12909-019-1764-y

37. Ullah, M., and Ameen, K. 2019. Teaching information literacy skills to medical students: perceptions of health sciences librarians. *Health Information and Libraries Journal*, 36(4), 357–66. https://doi.org/10.1111/hir.12279

38. Kingston, O., and Behjati, S. 2008. Academic medicine. *BMJ*, 336(7653), s172. https://doi.org/10.1136/bmj.39576.631238.CE

39. Jeffe, D.B., Andriole, D.A., Wathington, H.D., and Tai, R.H. 2014. The emerging physician-scientist workforce: demographic, experiential, and attitudinal predictors of MD-PhD program enrollment. *Academic Medicine*, 89(10), 1398–407. https://doi.org/10.1097/ACM.0000000000000400

40. O'Sullivan, P.S., Niehaus, B., Lockspeiser, T.M., and Irby, D.M. 2009. Becoming an academic doctor: perceptions of scholarly careers. *Medical Education*, 43(4), 335–41. https://doi.org/10.1111/j.1365-2923.2008.03270.x

41. Murdoch-Eaton, D., Drewery, S., Elton, S., Emmerson, C., Marshall, M., Smith, J.A., Stark, P., and Whittle, S. 2010. What do medical students understand by research and research skills? Identifying research opportunities within undergraduate projects. *Medical Teacher*, 32(3), e152–60. https://doi.org/10.3109/01421591003657493

42. Brown, L.M. 2020. See one, do one, teach one ... not anymore. *The Journal of Thoracic and Cardiovascular Surgery*, 159(6), 2497–8. https://doi.org/10.1016/j.jtcvs.2019.11.047

43. Rodriguez-Paz, J.M., Kennedy, M., Salas, E., Wu, A.W., Sexton, J.B., Hunt, E.A., and Pronovost, P.J. 2009. Beyond "see one, do one, teach one": toward a different training paradigm. *Quality and Safety in Health Care*, 18(1), 63. https://doi.org/10.1136/qshc.2007.023903

44. Nwomeh, B.C. 2012. Teaching technical skills to medical students: beyond "see one, do one, teach one." *Annals of African Medicine*, 11(1), 46–7. PMID: 22199048.

45. Erstad, B.L., and Stratton, T.P. 2021. Teaching ethics: see one, do one, … teach one? *American Journal of Pharmaceutical Education*, 86(2), ajpe8503. https://doi.org/10.5688/ajpe8503

46. Kotsis, S.V. and Chung, K.C. 2013. Application of the "see one, do one, teach one" concept in surgical training. *Plastic and Reconstructive Surgery*, 131(5), 1194–201. https://doi.org/10.1097/PRS.0b013e318287a0b3

47. Keren, D., Lockyer, J., and Ellaway, R.H. 2017. Social studying and learning among medical students: a scoping review. *Perspectives in Medical Education*, 6(5), 311–18. https://doi.org/10.1007/S40037-017-0358-9

48. Tannery, N.H., and Maggio, L.A. 2012. The role of medical librarians in medical education review articles. *Journal of the Medical Library Association*, 100(2), 142–4. https://doi.org/10.3163/1536-5050.100.2.015

49. Greyson, D., Surette, S., Dennett, L. and, Chatterley, T. 2013. "You're just one of the group when you're embedded": report from a mixed-method investigation of the research-embedded health librarian experience. *Journal of the Medical Library Association*, 101(4), 287–97. https://doi.org/10.3163/1536-5050.101.4.010

50. Ma, J., Stahl, L., and Knotts, E. 2018. Emerging roles of health information professionals for library and information science curriculum development: a scoping review. *Journal of the Medical Library Association*, 106(4), 432–44. https://doi.org/10.5195/jmla.2018.354

51. Ross-White, A. 2021. Search is a verb: systematic review searching as invisible labor. *Journal of the Medical Library Association*, 109(3), 505–6. https://doi.org/10.5195/jmla.2021.1226

13 "Your Favourite Conference Feels like Home Because Someone Is Doing the Housekeeping": How Conference Conveners Support Evidence-Informed Medical Education

LARA VARPIO, KATE MCOWEN, AND REENA KARANI

As a health professions education (HPE) researcher, conferences are important to me. Yes, they help me to stay on top of what's happening in the field, but there's so much more. When I go to certain HPE conferences, I honestly feel like I'm going home. I'm meeting my people – people who understand me and my research. I can change and grow in this community because that is – at its essence – what academics do: we conduct research to learn new things and we adjust our thinking to accommodate new knowledge. A good conference is where I can talk to my people about how my thinking is changing and how I'm growing. I learn how they're changing and growing too. We have history together. These are my peers, many of whom have become my friends. Like any home, these conferences are places where disagreement and heated debates happen, but the community is stronger for having aired our differences, examined the possibilities, and moved forward again with new or affirmed directions. When I go back to my private home, I'm rejuvenated and inspired thanks to the time spent in my academic home.

– Lara Varpio, Professor and Co-Director
of Research in Medical Education

Conferences fill my tank! As a teacher, medical education leader, and education scientist, my daily work is varied, harried, and challenging. I'm also always short-pressed for time. Conference participation affords me formal opportunities to learn, time to connect with colleagues and friends, and the space to reflect and rejuvenate. I'm also struck by what I leave conferences with: insightful learning aside, I always come back with new friends, exciting collaborations, the gift of perspectives shared by mentors, and the joy of new mentees. I feel renewed and energized. To me, my favourite conferences are like my home, and by "home" I mean more than a physical place. Connection and community are embodied in the word for me, and that is exactly how I feel about these experiences.

– Reena Karani, Professor and Director of The Institute
for Medical Education

We want delegates' conference experience to be amazing. We take it as a compliment – the highest form of praise, really – when delegates call our conference "home." We work really hard to make that happen. We know the program inside and out. We know what room each part of the program is happening in so that when a delegate is looking for a specific room, we can get them there quickly. We know the disaster protocols. If something goes wrong, we're ready. We are the ones running around behind the scenes to make sure everything runs smoothly and that small crises don't turn into big problems. We are the people who are always there, just present to be ready to step in, to support delegates, to be helpful. If delegates come to the conference for new knowledge, networking, and professional development, we are the ones making sure that these are their focus. We'll focus on keeping it all running. We'll make sure there's food, comfortable seating areas, and opportunities for great discussions. We are the organization's hosts. If delegates feel like the conference is home, it is our job to make that home welcoming. It is rewarding work, but it is also really hard. If we do our jobs well, delegates go home rejuvenated – but we'll go home exhausted.

– Kate McOwen, Senior Director of Medical Education Initiatives

Most of the people working in medical education who are celebrated in this book are co-located with medical learners – be that in the learning environments of the medical school or of clinical work contexts. However, there are also groups and individuals who are deeply involved in the medical education enterprise but who have minimal formal interaction with learners. One such group is the conveners of academic conferences that focus on medical education. In this chapter, we review the literature addressing the role of conferences in academia, highlight why these meetings are important to medical education, describe the role of conference convenors, and offer some reflections about why this work is worthy of more recognition in the field of medical education. In sum, this chapter celebrates these people who create spaces that feel like home.

   As an author team, this is a topic that touches very close to home. This is perhaps most true for Kate McOwen, who is the Senior Director of Educational and Student Affairs at the Association of American Medical Colleges (AAMC). In this position, Kate leads a unit responsible for the Association's external relationships with medical educators, administrators, scholars, student affairs leaders, advisors, and learners. Kate also leads the medical education and Research in Medical Education (RIME) calls for medical education submissions for the AAMC's annual Learn Serve Lead conference. Academic medicine's conference landscape is very much part of what Kate thinks about and reflects on in her daily professional work. Lara Varpio has worked extensively with Kate and the rest of the AAMC medical education team because, over the past 10 years, she has served on the Medical Education Planning committee, acting as chair of that committee for the past five years. Lara is a PhD-trained qualitative researcher who has worked in the field of health professions education since 2007 and has been consistently attending medical education academic meetings – both nationally and internationally – for over a decade. Reena is a geriatrician and palliative medicine physician and directs the Institute for Medical Education at the Icahn School of Medicine at Mount Sinai. She is an active presenter and contributor to medical education and specialty society academic meetings. Her engagement with the AAMC has included being a longstanding member of the Medical Education Planning committee, serving on the Learn Serve Lead planning committee and leading the RIME committee as chair. For our author team, conferences in medical education are important loci for our professional communities and our own careers.

The Role of Conferences in Academia

Academic meetings are typically arranged to bring researchers, educators, administrators, and other community members together to present and debate the latest research findings and the cutting-edge issues that are shaping a particular academic field. At these conferences, community members share knowledge and innovations with an audience of peers for real-time deliberation by and feedback from the community. Research suggests that the main motivations for attending academic conferences are to "get together to share information, interact, and to discuss matters of professional interest."[1] (p. 723) Academia is constantly evolving, offering new information and interventions that advance our ways of thinking about specific topics. To maintain awareness of and engagement in this development, academic communities rely – at least in part – on academic conferences.

While researchers and scholars working to advance a field of knowledge commonly rely on published peer-reviewed journal manuscripts, the structures of the publication process are slow to move. For an article to be published, it must pass through a gauntlet of editors and peer reviewers who can require several iterations of revise, resubmit, and re-review. By the time a manuscript is published in a journal, the data and insights therein are already outdated. In our personal experience, the fastest timeline between submission and publication is six months. The longest was four times as long.

Therefore, to access the most recent ideas and knowledge that are being developed around the world, academic community members rely on informal, not-yet-published dissemination venues. The most actively used of these venues is the academic meeting or conference.[2] Conference submissions are typically peer-reviewed, meaning that the content presented in the meeting has been vetted by select members of the community and judged to be of high quality. Furthermore, the turnaround time from submission to presentation is usually less than 12 months. This means that conference presentations offer rigorous insights from work that scholars are currently conducting. Thus, the conference is a space where exchanges of up-to-date ideas and knowledge can happen. Given the concentration of scholars at the conference, these meetings also attract industry representatives, organizational bodies, funding agency delegates, and others who want to learn about the latest advances in the field, and who want to network with community members for their own purposes.

But conferences do more than just support the development and dissemination of knowledge. Research suggests that conferences serve important social functions as well. Different studies have confirmed that the success of an individual's academic career is dependent – in a variety of ways – on the extent to which that person is part of research networks.[3–5] In other words, part of an individual academic's success is contingent on their position within the field's community network, and the degree of influence they have because of that position.[6] In a parallel body of work, research has also suggested that being in close proximity with other scholars gives rise to serendipity-based generation of ideas, allows for implicit methodological knowledge to be shared, and creates opportunity for latent ideas to be solidified through mutual in-person discussions among experts.[7] Therefore, to engage in, manoeuvre within, and harness the power of these networks, individual scholars attend academic conferences where they can meet new and existing colleagues. While the merits of virtual versus in-person meetings continue to be debated across academia,[8–10] academic conferences are still considered essential events that exist at the forefront of scientific and professional development.[8,11]

The beneficial interpersonal aspects of academic conferences are also tied to the professional identity development and socialization functions of these meetings. Research suggests that individual members of an academic community are acknowledged as members of the community and positioned in the field's social order through their engagement in different events, like conferences.[12] In academic meetings, scholars engage with each other "not only as researchers who represent intellectual claims, but also as colleagues. In so doing, they attribute not only intellectual statements, but also social identities and roles to one another."[12] (p. 922) Being recognized as a scholar of importance at a conference – e.g., by being invited to give the keynote lecture – allows individual members of the academic community to negotiate an appropriate salary, supervise learners, take on leadership roles, and participate in decision-making panels.[12] In these ways, and others, visibility at an academic conference has impact across many aspects of a scholar's life – including the accumulation of status, resources, and power.[1,12] To summarize, "conferences are complex events that shape the working lives of academics."[13] (p. 86)

The Role of Conferences in Medical Education

While the aforementioned purposes are met in medical education conferences, our conferences have additional important functions. For instance, medical education conferences are spaces where a unique kind of community building takes place. The medical education continuum (undergraduate, graduate, and continuing medical education [UME, GME, CME]) comprises many different groups of people; however, there is often only one person from each group at any one institution. For example, in most medical schools or teaching hospitals, there is one person who heads up student affairs, a different person leading accreditation, and another individual directing the education research unit. When those individuals face challenges or unexpected experiences, they often do not have a colleague within their local context to turn to for advice, ideas, solutions, or solace. In the absence of local colleagues, many people who are essential to the running of UME, GME, and CME need to have ties to peers in the same role at other institutions. How do they make these connections? Often during special sessions at medical education conferences that are designed specifically for a particular subgroup in the community – e.g., at the closed meeting of student affairs leaders; at special sessions for program administrators; at the forum about accreditation visits that is given a special space in the conference program; at the by-invitation meeting of directors of medical education research units. It is in these special streams of the conference program that subgroup communities are fostered.

The vital importance of these subgroup communities was made keenly evident during the COVID-19 pandemic. During that crisis, individual institutions needed to quickly learn from the successes and failures at other medical schools and teaching hospitals. Student affairs leaders informally turned to their network of colleagues for solutions to the unprecedented problems that suddenly needed to be resolved.

Individuals leading accreditation preparations needed to unofficially liaise with peers at other institutions to figure out how to successfully hold virtual accreditation visits. Directors of education research units relied on their professional network to create ways for maintaining scholarly programs of work when medical schools and teaching hospitals were not allowing non-essential personnel to go to work. These professional networks allowed individuals to quickly learn from each other across institutions. Anecdotal evidence suggests that these relationships were essential to finding ways to continue to train healthcare professionals during truly unprecedented times.

Conferences are important meetings where these subgroups can find colleagues and peers, and where they can learn from each other's successes and failures. Medical education can be a lonely field – e.g., at a medical school, there might be *one* assessment and evaluation researcher, *one* assistant dean of equity, diversity, and inclusion, *one* admissions leader. These individuals regularly rely on their community of peers. To be part of that community, these individuals come together at the academic conferences to grow relationships and, in so doing, grow ties that can help improve medical education at many institutions. As this example from Kate's experiences illustrates, medical education conference convenors have frequently heard stories of the importance of these networks from meeting delegates:

> *I've had occasions where I'm sitting in a restaurant with another member of the conference convening team and have someone come running up to me whom I didn't recognize who said:*
>
> *"I don't know if you remember me, but you ran this speed networking event at a meeting a few years ago and I ended up at a table with a whole group of people I didn't know from all over the nation. We were all [topic X] deans and we were concerned about [topic X] and we formed a special interest group. We studied the problem across our many institutions. Because of what we've learned, we've made important, beneficial changes at our local institutions. None of this would have ever happened if it hadn't been for that networking session at the conference. We wouldn't have had these successes without you."*
>
> *That's one of the things that's special about medical education meetings. We give people a chance to meet their peers from other institutions. We make medical education a little less lonely for them.*

Another purpose of a medical education conference is to create a space for wrestling with our field's most difficult problems. Some organizations make the decision to hold time in their conferences to have topic-focused events – be it networking sessions, symposia, or other program offerings – where people from a range of different roles in the field come together to address a particularly wicked problem[13] that is hampering the HPE community's success. At medical education conferences, individuals have the chance to step away from the day-to-day demands of their careers to examine the challenges and opportunities of the field. They can meet with people who work in very different aspects of the medical education continuum but who are working on the same wicked problem. At the meeting, in these parts of the program that are dedicated to different topics or goals, individuals can cross-pollinate – across institutions, across roles within the same institution, across UME/GME/CME divisions – to learn from each other, to work together, or even just to commiserate. In fact, sometimes it is at these meetings that individuals within *the same institution* can learn of progress being made on challenges they are facing. These focused parts of the conference program are, as Kate explains, an important part of medical education meetings:

> *I was at a meeting that we had convened focused on a particular topic and a delegate from one a very large institution – one of the many institutions present at the meeting – came up to me and said:*
>
> *"I just have to tell you that I was sitting at the table and met a person who was very engaging and thoughtful. They told me about their research and their work in their institution and I was fascinated. I was so excited about their ideas and their approaches. I asked them what school they were from – and they're from my school! I had no idea! I had worked at that school for 20 years and the other person had been there even longer, and we had never met before. We are engaged in the same effort at the same institution, but we had never crossed paths."*

The Role of Conference Conveners

For medical education conferences to meet all these purposes, it takes a team of people who work tirelessly to bring these conferences to life. These convenors are involved in every aspect of the meeting, working to ensure that every minute of the program is filled with the most useful, productive, important, and informative sessions possible. They arrange for the peer review of hundreds (if not thousands) of abstract, poster, and workshop submissions to ensure that each receives due consideration. They lead several committees of volunteer community members who appraise the submissions and associated peer review comments to select which submissions will be given time in the conference program. They work with community members to decide which special sessions, closed meetings, and events will be held to address the needs of individual affinity groups. They construct a conference program trying to ensure that communities with similar interests are not scheduled against each other, that individual speakers aren't booked to be in two places at once, and that the richest diversity of voices possible are present at the meeting. They consider national and international perspectives about what are the most pressing concerns and mandates for the field to address. And they balance all these considerations with the priorities, mandates, and expectations of the organization that funds the conference. Clearly the role of conference convenor is full of complex work and decision-making.

And yet, while conference convenors are part of every aspect of a conference, they have little power over the conference program itself. But, since they are *the face* of the conference, conveners are the ones who receive all delegate feedback. Conferences are important to the medical education field and the individuals who work therein, and so feedback about the conference is equally important – but sometimes there is nothing a convener can do to address concerns. For instance, at the level of individual conference attendees, having your submission accepted for presentation at a conference is considered a piece of evidence of the impact of your work. It is acknowledged and considered by local promotion and tenure committees. Individuals' careers are truly impacted by the opinions of conference submission reviewers and the decisions of conference program committees. But it is the convenors who have the responsibility of informing each submitter if their work was accepted or denied for podium time, poster space, or workshop time. While the power of making those decisions is largely not in the hands of the conveners, they are tasked to be the messengers of the decisions. Time and again, it is the conveners who receive backlash from submitters who were not accepted into the conference program.

Conference conveners also work hard to ensure that any one individual is not over-represented on the conference program. They cross check and double check the program in an effort to increase the diversity of individuals who are awarded time in the conference program. And yet, since no system is perfect, some individuals are inevitably present on the program several times. And who hears the complaints that so-and-so is getting preferential treatment or is podium-hogging? The conveners.

There are also dozens of affinity groups who want to have time and space set aside in the conference program. And yet, the program itself is finite – there are only so many days, so many rooms, and so much capacity in each room. This means that not every group will be able to be given dedicated time and space in the program. Every year, someone complains that their group was not recognized as sufficiently "special" to merit a dedicated space, but that they are in fact very special indeed. Guess who hears those criticisms.

Concluding Thoughts

Medical education's conference conveners are thoughtful, committed, and passionate individuals who spend their time working to create meetings that respect and serve the many perspectives, identities, roles, and needs of the *entire* medical education community. When their efforts are successful, delegates can focus on their goals for the meeting. They meet peers, gain new knowledge, network within the community, and build important professional relationships. As research describes[13] and as our own experiences confirm, conference participants often describe their preferred meeting as their *academic home*.[13] If a conference achieves that status, it is the conference conveners that do the housework so that the conference house feels like a welcoming home.[13]

We call on the medical education community to recognize the work of the conference convener. It is thanks to their labour that we are able to harness these meetings for all of the purposes we bring to that space. As Kate's reflection highlights, their work is often uncelebrated but without them the meetings would not be home:

The staff who work behind the scenes of medical education's conferences strive to construct an event that brings together the full array of interests that are part of our medical education community. They work humbly and passionately. They work with members of the community to make consequential decisions to shape the conference, but they do so from a position of support. The convener staff are committed, brilliant, innovative changemakers who are dedicated to supporting the medical education community.

We also hope that each member of the medical education community remembers the dedication and generosity of spirit that conveners have so that when feedback is offered, it is shared in the same spirit. Kate further notes:

I wish people understood that the convenors who pull together these conferences do so for the professional development of others and to nurture the rich and varied discourse of our field. There is no personal gain for them. I wish people understood just how selfless the staff conveners are. It is our job to take in all the compliments and all the complaints – to assess it, learn from it, and make the next conference offering even better. I just wish people would remember that we care deeply about the content and the community when they come up to us and give us feedback.

The work undertaken by conference convenors is to make academic homes for all of us in medical education. We ask all members of the community to join us in appreciating and applauding the work of these homemakers.

Additional Reading

Burford, J., Bosanquet, A., and Smith, J. 2020. "Homeliness meant having the fucking vacuum cleaner out": the gendered labour of maintaining conference communities. *Gender and Education*, 32(1), 86–100. https://doi.org/10.1080/09540253.2019.1680809

Kroll, H., and Neuhäusler, P. 2022. "Formal and informal networkedness among German Academics": exploring the role of conferences and co-publications in scientific performance. *Scientometrics*, 127, 6431–52. https://doi.org/10.1007/s11192-022-04526-z

Rowe, N. 2018. "When you get what you want, but not what you need": the motivations, affordances and shortcomings of attending academic/scientific conferences. *International Journal of Research in Education and Science*, 4(2), 714–29. https://doi.org/10.21890/ijres.438394

References

1. Rowe, N. 2018. "When you get what you want, but not what you need": the motivations, affordances and shortcomings of attending academic/scientific conferences. *International Journal of Research in Education and Science*, 4(2), 714–29. https://doi.org/10.21890/ijres.438394

2. Hauss, K. 2021. What are the social and scientific benefits of participating at academic conferences? Insights from a survey among doctoral students and postdocs in Germany. *Research Evaluation*, 30(1), 1–2. https://doi.org/10.1093/reseval/rvaa018

3. Abbasi, A., Altmann, J., and Hossain, L. 2011. Identifying the effects of co-authorship networks on the performance of scholars: a correlation and regression analysis of performance measures and social network analysis measures. *Journal of Informatics*, 5(4), 594–607. https://doi.org/10.1016/j.joi.2011.05.007

4. Abbasi, A., Hossain, L., and Leydesdorff, L. 2012. Betweenness centrality as a driver of preferential attachment in the evolution of research collaboration networks. *Journal of Informatics*, 6(3), 403–12. https://doi.org/10.1016/j.joi.2012.01.002

5. Guan, J., Yan, Y., and Zhang, J. 2015. How do collaborative features affect scientific output? Evidences from wind power field. *Scientometrics*, 102(1), 333–55. https://doi.org/10.1007/s11192-014-1311-x

6. Xu, Q., and Chang, V. 2020. Analysis of co-authorship network and the correlation between academic performance and social network measures. In *5th International Conference on Internet of Things, Big Data and Security (IoTBDS)*, pp. 359–66. SciTePress. https://doi.org/10.1016/j.iot.2020.100307

7. Kroll, H., and Neuhäusler, P. 2022. "Formal and informal networkedness among German academics": exploring the role of conferences and co-publications in scientific performance. *Scientometrics*, 127, 6431–52. https://doi.org/10.1007/s11192-022-04526-z

8. Donjon, E. 2021. Lost and found: the academic conference in pandemic and post-pandemic times. *Irish Educational Studies*, 40(2), 367–73. https://doi.org/10.1080/03323315.2021.1932554

9. Goebel, J., Manion, C., Millei, Z., Read, R., and Silova, I. 2020. Academic conferencing in the age of COVID-19 and climate crisis: the case of the Comparative and International Education Society (CIES). *International Review of Education*, 66, 797–816. https://doi.org/10.1007/s11159-020-09873-8

10. Chalvatzis, K., and Ormosi, P.L. 2021. The carbon impact of flying to economics conferences: is flying more associated with more citations? *Journal of Sustainable Tourism*, 29(1), 40–67. https://doi.org/10.1080/09669582.2020.1806858

11. Seidenberg, N., Scheffel, M., Kovanovic, V., Lynch, G., and Drachsler, H. 2021. Virtual academic conferences as learning spaces: factors associated with the perceived value of purely virtual conferences. *Journal of Computer Assisted Learning*, 37(6), 1694–707. https://doi.org/10.1111/jcal.12614

12. Hamann, J. 2019. The making of professors: assessment and recognition in academic recruitment. *Social Studies of Science*, 49(6), 919–41. https://doi.org/10.1177/0306312719880017

13. Burford, J., Bosanquet, A., and Smith, J. 2020. 'Homeliness meant having the fucking vacuum cleaner out': the gendered labour of maintaining conference communities. *Gender and Education*, 32(1), 86–100. https://doi.org/10.1080/09540253.2019.1680809

14. Rittel, H., Webber, W.J., and Melvin, M. 1973. Dilemmas in a general theory of planning. *Policy Sciences*, 4(2), 155–69. https://doi.org/10.1007/BF01405730

14 Ghostwriting Grants: A Critical Conversation about the Invisible Contributors to Health Professions Education Research Grants

JACQUELINE TORTI, MARIAM HAYWARD,
FARAH FRIESEN, AND LORELEI LINGARD

No researcher writes their grants alone.[1] Think about the last time you submitted a medical education research grant. Recall the cast of players involved in pulling it together: the clinicians, educators, scientists, graduate students, research staff, librarians, university research administrators, and subject-matter experts. Think of all the intellectual work: conceptualizing the problem, strengthening the rationale, designing the methods, selecting the sample, articulating clear objectives and outcomes. Remember all the technical and organizational steps: coordinating the team's work, observing the funder's eligibility and formatting requirements, securing signatures and support letters, designing effective visuals, double-checking the budget numbers.

Now, visualize the list of investigator names on the front sheet of that grant. Who was there? And, more to the point for our chapter, who was not? Likely all the contributors who were *not* faculty were missing from the investigator list. The graduate students, the research assistants, the university staff, the librarians – these are the ghostwriters behind our grants. Their essential work is neither acknowledged nor represented. Why is this the case? And what is the impact? This chapter will unearth some of the "on-the-ground" practices and processes of grant writing to critically examine how current structures instigate invisibility.

We are an authorship team with lived experience of this invisible work and the structures that produce it. Jacqueline Torti spent five years between her PhD and her first faculty position in research staff roles, trying to support faculty projects while keeping her own scholarly momentum. Mariam Hayward is a first-generation student born in Kabul, Afghanistan with more than 20 years' experience of program management, research design and implementation, mixed-methods evaluation, grant-writing development, knowledge exchange, and research administration in the university setting;

she is currently Director, Inclusive Research Excellence and Impact at Western University. Farah Friesen is trained as a librarian with a Master of Information and brings her experience of more than eight years in a research staff role; she is currently Manager, Research & Knowledge Mobilization at the University of Toronto's Centre for Advancing Collaborative Healthcare & Education (CACHE) at University Health Network. Lorelei Lingard brings to this chapter more than two decades of experience with leading grants, mentoring graduate students to develop their grantsmanship, collaborating with academic staff in specialized roles, and chairing or participating in grant review panels. Through a series of conversations about our various perspectives and experiences, we decided to weave our main messages into a set of three dilemmas that we present and critically analyse in this chapter.

Grant capture is integral to one's academic and professional career. A track record in grant capture influences promotions and tenure, awards and distinctions, continued research agendas, career trajectories, and future opportunities. Being named on a grant has social and financial implications as it confers credit, identifies valued contributions, and can validate expertise. Yet the literature on grant writing is both limited and narrowly oriented. In health professions education (HPE) and other academic fields, the literature focuses on how to write a grant and successfully obtain research funding, with emphasis on issues such as developing a robust research question.[2-7] Because grants are necessary for promotions and recognition in academic institutions, there is also attention to interventions and structural facilitators that improve grant-writing skills.[8-11]

The current literature is instructional rather than critical: it focuses on how to play the grant-writing game rather than questioning the way the game is played. What is missing is critical literature on grant writing that moves beyond skills to consider the social processes of establishing, leading, and working as part of a grant-writing team. What has received some critical attention is the peer review process of grants[12,13] and the impact of current grant funding structures on research integrity. However, reducing professional ethics to individual integrity is problematic as it ignores structural policies (e.g., promotions criteria) that might inadvertently encourage certain practices.[14-17] Conix et al.[18] have argued that current funding systems incentivize questionable behaviours that might lead researchers to violate moral values according to Merton's Code of Conduct of accountability, honesty, impartiality, responsibility, and fairness. These values have practical effects on research integrity, such as the fabrication or falsification of data, mitigating risk and harm to participants, and respecting and acknowledging the work of others.

Missing from the limited body of critical work on grant peer review and research integrity is attention to issues of grant authorship. This gap is somewhat surprising, given the extensive attention to the adjacent issue of manuscript authorship. Literature within and beyond HPE explores questionable research practices, including authorship issues such as honorary (gift) authorship, ghost authorship, and authorship order.[19-25] However, the literature characterizes authorship dilemmas as matters of individual choice rather than examining the structures that incentivize and reward behaviour. While insights from the manuscript authorship literature have some relevance, grant writing presents unique challenges that deserve focused attention.

Dilemmas That Produce Invisibility

This section critically addresses the power and politics of grant writing by examining three dilemmas that produce invisibility: choosing career or contract, gaming eligibility, and institutionalizing invisibility.

Box 1. Dilemma 1: Choosing Career or Contract

Yoni sits down to have a mentorship conversation around grant authorship with their supervisor. Yoni aspires to a future faculty role and is currently contracted to work as a research associate to help build up their curriculum vitae (CV). Yoni needs to make a difficult decision about the grant they are currently preparing: be named as an investigator in recognition of their intellectual input or be paid from the budget as a research associate. Yoni's supervisor helps sort through the considerations based on their academic goals and economic needs. In the end, Yoni and their supervisor decide it is best to set up Yoni to be paid out of the grant, securing extended employment as a research associate. Yoni still contributes intellectually to the grant but as a ghostwriter rather than a named investigator, trading academic recognition for economic security.

What Creates This Dilemma?

Research associates who aspire to future academic faculty positions are regularly confronted with this dilemma in the Canadian funding context. This dilemma arises because of eligibility rules governing who can be listed as an investigator on grant applications. With few exceptions, individuals need an academic appointment to be listed as the principal investigator (PI) or co-investigator (Co-I) on a grant application. For most contract research associates, this eligibility rule automatically excludes them regardless of the extent of their intellectual contribution to the grant proposal. Adjunct appointments may offer a workaround: these are honorific, non-remunerated, and limited-term appointments. This workaround, however, does not address the second eligibility rule underpinning this dilemma, which dictates who can be paid from a grant. Because most Canadian funders do not allow investigators to be paid from the grant, research associates will need to choose between being named as an investigator and being employed.

Why Does This Dilemma Matter?

This dilemma highlights the vulnerability and invisibility of individuals in contract research roles when they participate in grant writing. The implications could be profound for those aspiring to a future faculty appointment. Regardless of the degree of their intellectual contribution or leadership role in a grant proposal, they can realize that contribution in terms of what Bourdieu[26] calls "symbolic capital" (access to resources based on recognition and prestige) or "economic capital" (material assets like money), but not both. And the more often this choice is made, the more the die is cast: faculty with higher symbolic capital are positioned to accrue more resources, including more symbolic and economic capital.[27,28] Advantage begets more advantage: the named investigator's CV will gradually build, strengthening their chances at the faculty roles they're applying for and future income gains. At the same time, the contract researcher's CV will suggest an increasing detour from the linear pathway between graduate training and faculty appointment.

In light of this, "choice" oversimplifies Yoni's situation. This dilemma is not about individual choice: it is about the structural reproduction of invisibility and inequity. Invisibility because Yoni's decision to be paid from rather than named on the grant means that their intellectual work is invisible both to the funder and future potential employers. And inequity because economic need is influenced by gender, race, income, and other social demographics.[29-32] In our example, Yoni could be a 39-year-old single mother of two or a 27-year-old male living at home: these individuals are not equitably impacted by the eligibility rules. The latter may be able to "choose" symbolic over economic capital; the former with her additional single-parent responsibilities may not. Given that women are more likely than men to be employed casually between PhD and faculty appointment,[33] this dilemma reinforces systematic inequity and undermines efforts to increase diversity of early-career faculty.[34–36]

If we acknowledge that these dilemmas are not merely about difficult individual choices, we need to explicitly discuss the structures that produce – and reproduce – them. One of these structures is the apprenticeship model of research training, where many learn grant-writing skills and practices.[37] Yoni's supervisor makes the eligibility dilemma an explicit, strategic conversation, but other supervisors might not. Another supervisor might assume that Yoni, the single mother, needs the contract appointment and, therefore, not even suggest the adjunct professor workaround to the eligibility rule. Or a supervisor might assume that Yoni will work on the grant application but not be named, using the eligibility rule to enforce a tradition of "paying your dues" as a junior member of the research team. This assumption is not unlikely given the "postdoc bottleneck"[38] (p. 354) in academia, where the supply of PhD-trained researchers may exceed demand in some disciplines and/or national contexts. Such a "labour-excess economy" has been criticized for producing a "legion of the discontented";[39] (p. 1105) we would argue that it also sustains a legion of the disenfranchised, in which individuals like Yoni are vulnerable to expectations that they pay their dues because, if they do not, another underemployed PhD or postdoc will. Such scenarios reveal the profound influence of such supervisory assumptions, which often remain tacit in communications about grant authorship. Therefore, rather than uncritical adherence to eligibility criteria, critical conversations need to take place among the research teams preparing grants.[1,40] If not, Yoni risks unconsciously reproducing their own experiences when they become a supervisor.[37,39]

Box 2. Dilemma 2: Gaming Eligibility

Thomas is a young early-career PhD scientist in an HPE research centre. He is in his annual mentorship committee meeting, and the committee is discussing his emerging profile as a researcher. Committee members have commented that two of his large grants have him listed as a co-investigator, and they are concerned that he is not developing his role as a lead investigator. Thomas explains that he is leading the project; the order of investigators is just an eligibility workaround because these funders require a physician to be the PI on the grant. The committee members warn that this pattern on the funding section of Thomas' CV could be problematic for promotion and tenure.

What Creates This Dilemma?

Funding eligibility criteria do not stop at requiring a faculty appointment: they may also dictate that named applicants meet other criteria, such as specific degrees, affiliations, or memberships. For example, medical organizations (such as the Physician Services Incorporated Foundation) require principal applicants to be "a College of Physicians and Surgeons of Ontario licensed MD," and professional organizations (such as the Canadian Association of Medical Education or the Association of Medical Education in Europe) restrict applications to members. Faced with these requirements, applicants like Thomas can either not apply for funding from these organizations or resort to gaming eligibility. Thomas takes the latter path: he names as PI another member of the research team who meets the funder's criteria that the PI must be a physician. Perhaps the named PI will substantially contribute to the grant and fulfil the role of principal (or co-principal) investigator. But if they do not, if it is their title that does the heavy lifting, with others taking the lead role but not receiving credit, then we have a situation of invisible work.

Why Does This Dilemma Matter?

When gaming eligibility happens, what is at stake is legitimacy. In Thomas' case, as a non-physician, he has no legitimacy in this funder's eyes: he must borrow that legitimacy at the cost of sacrificing his position as named PI. Legitimacy is not inherent: physicians are not inevitably more legitimate in funders' eyes than PhDs; sometimes quite the opposite. Legitimacy is constructed by the funder's eligibility criteria. For Thomas' current funder, the MD has legitimacy but the PhD does not. But other funders assign legitimacy differently. Thomas could be a community-academic physician who works as a clinical educator with an adjunct appointment at a medical school. He is on an academic career path and seeking funding for his research, but he does not have the type of appointment he needs to be eligible to apply for other kinds of grants such as a Social Sciences and Humanities Research grant with the Canadian Tri-Council funding agency. In this case, the clinical status is not recognized as legitimate, and accessing this funding opportunity would require gaming. For instance, Thomas could collaborate with a full-time faculty member who could serve as PI on their grant to satisfy the eligibility criteria.

Such eligibility workarounds involve gifting the role of the PI to access a funding opportunity. This can take various forms; the shared characteristic, however, is that the work of the actual author(s) is not accurately acknowledged. Gaming eligibility through gifting PI roles is a common but unspoken practice – a "public secret."[18] (p. 6) The practice arises in response to structural conditions that, according to Conix and colleagues,[18] strongly incentivize researchers to violate authorship norms and the ethical principles of honesty and fairness. Such practices matter not only because of the ethical questions they raise but also because of their ripple effects in the granting system. As Anderson and colleagues have argued, funding structures such as eligibility requirements "may lead scientists to be strategic in ways that contradict traditional normative cultures in science"[41] (p. 858) and "skew this system in unanticipated and perverse ways, with negative consequences for science as well as for the lives and careers of scientists."[42] (p. 438)

We conceptualize gaming eligibility as a dilemma because it is a logical strategy under the circumstances, yet it produces unanticipated and perverse effects. First, gifting PI status simultaneously creates and limits opportunity: it creates the potential for funding success but also penalizes those who made the intellectual contributions behind the scenes. This penalty expands beyond the loss of status on a particular grant because "receiving research grants is among the highlights of an academic career, affirming previous accomplishments and enabling new research endeavours."[15] (p. 4441) Thus, the penalty is cumulative, affecting both recognition of input on this grant and opportunities downstream. Second, gifting PI status can, ironically, take away opportunities from the named PI if the research team assumes that the named PI's role is *only* gifted and fails to meaningfully engage them in the work. If their participation is thus restricted, they will not meet the qualifications for authorship on publications arising from the research, potentially creating an asymmetry on their CV. Thus, approaching the practice of gaming eligibility *as a dilemma* highlights that what starts as an apparently simple, pragmatic decision – gift the PI role to the eligible team member – can have career implications for all involved.

Box 3. Dilemma 3: Institutionalizing Invisibility

Theresa is preparing her CV for a job application and is trying to find evidence to describe the depth of her contributions to grant writing in her staff role as an equity, diversity, and inclusion (EDI) specialist. Theresa supports faculty members in thinking through how to integrate these aspects as part of their research programs, projects, and grants. Meaningful integration often means Theresa's contributions go well beyond technical and administrative support and are most accurately characterized as conceptual and intellectual contributions that shape the research questions and proposed activities, influencing the direction of the research. Despite these contributions, both Theresa's staff role and granting agency policies preclude her from being named on grants. Theresa now finds it challenging to describe her contributions and impacts within these grants as she embarks on the next step in her career journey.

What Creates This Dilemma?

Higher education institutions have long held central offices designed to support research through a suite of administrative services.[43] Traditionally, these research administrative roles have existed separate from academic and teaching roles. However, in recent years, there has been a rise in "third space professionals" or "para-academic roles" that exist between academic and professional spheres, such as equity roles like the one held by Theresa.[44-45] Many higher education institutions have created staff roles among these central research offices to support unique areas of increasing emphasis within the research funding landscape, such as knowledge translation or mobilization, EDI, decolonization, and Indigenization. These newer roles have a greater focus on research development than their administrative forebears. They are intended to provide subject-matter expertise to maximize researchers' success in representing these increasingly important aspects in their research and increasing the competitiveness of grant applications while advancing social justice and societal outcomes.[46]

The support offered by these specialized roles goes beyond the historical view of administrators as "guardians of the regulations" where contributions are devalued to administrative and clerical tasks;[47 (p. 133)] instead, these individuals can drive the direction of the research, infused across the proposed activities. Across many national and international research funding landscapes, these specialized areas (such as EDI) are increasingly weighed in evaluating grant applications, and investigators are increasingly seeking input from individuals in these staff roles. Individuals like Theresa meet with the core research team to discuss the research, conceptualize feasible and impactful methods, and review and write grant sections to embed language and concrete practices and strategies, as well as to ensure integration into the proposed activities that both meet evaluation criteria and have a clear linkage to outcomes and impacts.[48] But these contributions are invisible, as Theresa and specialized staff like her are not commonly named on the grant applications they support.

Why Does This Dilemma Matter?

This invisibility is the consequence of institutional design and funding agency parameters around named roles on grant applications, both of which exclude research staff from being named on grant applications. The consequences of this dilemma are multiple: it fosters an underappreciation of the contributions made by individuals in these staff roles; perpetuates unrecognized expertise that limits the credibility of these individuals as subject-matter experts; and creates downstream inequities as individuals in these roles struggle to provide evidence of their contributions when applying for promotions, awards, or professional growth opportunities.

Understanding knowledge and expertise and where they reside is a complex issue exacerbated in higher education institutions by the introduction of specialized roles in the research administration landscape. The polarization of non-academic (or staff) and academic roles can be argued to have led to inequity in how institutions recognize and credit knowledge generation and expertise. The knowledge that staff lend to their roles is often viewed as owned by the institution, which contrasts with academic positions that are credited and recognized with individual expertise. Institutional policies and practices need to be revisited, recognizing the merging or blurring of non-academic and academic roles in these specialized staff roles.[49] Higher education research offices have refocused work from mainly administrative functions to roles that contribute skills, knowledge, and value that are intellectual (rather than technical). This work and these contributions blur and challenge boundaries between administrators and academics.[43,46,50]

This invisibility dilemma is further compounded by funding agency definitions of co-applicant and collaborator, where such roles are designated for individuals who are expected to actively participate in proposed activities or provide a specialized service. Implicit in these definitions is the prioritization of contributions to the implementation of proposed research activities over conceptual contributions that led to the proposed research activities, including those conducted by integral community partners.[51] One possible explanation is that, historically, those involved in the conceptualization were the same as those involved in the implementation. But with the rise of "third space professions" or "para-academics," these definitions – and the preferential recognition of those involved in research execution – render some of those involved in conceptualization invisible. As Musselin[52] suggests, academic and non-academic work are becoming closer: as the distance between academic and staff roles diminishes, so should customs and regulations governing recognition of staff contributions evolve.

Concluding Thoughts

We are in a historical moment when the field of HPE is increasingly critically reflective about the authorship of publications but less attentive to the authorship of grants. This chapter attempts to address this gap by elucidating three dilemmas that produce invisibility in grant writing at individual and structural levels: forcing a "choice" of symbolic capital (career) or economic capital (contract); gaming eligibility; and institutionalizing invisibility where those in specialized staff roles do not have the ability to have their contributions appropriately recognized. While certain characters star in each dilemma, the dilemmas intersect and can be experienced regardless of role (e.g., Dilemma 1 could apply as much to a staff member as a graduate student). We recognize that this is not an exhaustive list of dilemmas; one unexamined is how to recognize administrative contributions to grants (e.g., project coordination and management).

We have demonstrated that these dilemmas produce invisibility in multiple ways. Additionally, we wish to point out that *the dilemmas themselves are largely invisible* because they contravene explicit codes and can be construed as "unethical." For instance, we all know that postdocs write the grants that employ them without receiving due credit. We both accept this practice and understand that it is bad form to discuss it. And who is in a position to critique when all are culpable to varying degrees? Thus, these dilemmas remain silent, unstudied, and continuously reproduced as HPE researchers learn their grant writing through apprenticeship.

Furthermore, the invisibility of these invisibilities risks the continued framing of these grant-writing concerns as issues of individual choice. We hope these dilemmas illustrate the problems with this framing and spotlight the misalignment between current structures and desirable (e.g., ethical, individual) practices. Only when we call attention to these as structural, political dilemmas rather than individual, moral ones will we begin to recognize and, hopefully, dismantle the structures and practices that (re)produce them. In this spirit, we close this chapter with recommendations for individuals and institutions.

Recommendations for Individuals

1. Awareness. We know that each of these dilemmas is experienced in HPE, but we also know these dilemmas are largely invisible. A key recommendation for individuals is to be aware (and to admit) that these dilemmas exist.
2. Conversation. Have explicit and upfront conversations with the research team about the different roles individuals will play in the grant-writing process and how those will be recognized and acknowledged in the grant application and throughout the research project.
3. Advocacy. It is not sufficient just to be aware and to have conversations about the invisible work around grant writing; we need to begin to resist some of these assumptions and advocate for visibility for ourselves and others.

Recommendations for Institutions and Funders

Having individuals confront these dilemmas differently is important but insufficient. Structural efforts are paramount.

1. Improvise. Institutions should take eligibility dilemmas seriously. Instead of invoking "the eligibility rules" and turning a blind eye (or even encouraging) the practice of gifting PI status, institutions can be more creative about offering people titles or adjuncts to navigate funders' eligibility criteria.
2. Reimagine. Funders should critically revisit eligibility criteria which create elite groups with access to funds and disenfranchise groups that do not. With the focus on community or industry research and partnerships with industry, the requirement for a university appointment to access many national funds is outdated and beginning to be reimagined. Many non-profit and Indigenous-led organizations can now apply for funding; such creative reimagining should also extend to other groups, sectors, and partners. Additionally, attention should be paid to rethinking co-applicant and collaborator roles to recognize conceptual contributions.
3. Be transparent. Institutions should create transparent decision processes, such as when to improvise about titles/roles, considerations for research staff to be named on grants, or how to recognize when research staff contribute conceptually to grant design. As we improvise and reimagine, responding creatively to

grant structures and requirements, transparency will ensure that opportunities are equitably distributed and contributions made visible.

4. Decolonize. Institutions' differential valuing of various forms of grant contributions perpetuates inequities. In this age of interdisciplinary research collaboration and community partnerships, the traditional hierarchy of placing most of the value on the PI needs dismantling. Furthermore, the gender and racial dimensions of the dilemmas we have discussed demand critical attention to the social value we implicitly attach to certain identities, titles, and roles, resulting in differential funding access.

Additional Reading

Cline, H., Coolen, L., de Vries, S., Hyman, S., Segal, R., and Steward, O. 2020. Recognizing team science contributions in academic hiring, promotion, and tenure. *The Journal of Neuroscience*, 40(35), 6662. https://doi.org/10.1523/JNEUROSCI.1139-20.2020

Conix, S., De Block, A., and Vaesen, K. 2021. Grant writing and grant peer review as questionable research practices. *F1000Research*, 10, 1126. https://doi.org/10.12688/f1000research.73893.2

Whitchurch, C. 2012. *Reconstructing Identities in Higher Education: The Rise of Third Space Professionals*. Routledge.

References

1. Cline, H., Coolen, L., de Vries, S., Hyman, S., Segal, R., and Steward, O. 2020. Recognizing team science contributions in academic hiring, promotion, and tenure. *The Journal of Neuroscience*, 40(35), 6662. https://doi.org/10.1523/JNEUROSCI.1139-20.2020

2. Blanco, M.A., and Lee, M.Y. 2012. Twelve tips for writing educational research grant proposals. *Medical Teacher*, 34(6), 450–3. https://doi.org/10.3109/0142159X.2012.668246

3. Wisdom, J.P., Riley, H., and Myers, N. 2015. Recommendations for writing successful grant proposals: an information synthesis. *Academic Medicine*, 90(12), 1720–5. https://doi.org/10.1097/ACM.0000000000000811

4. Blanco, M.A., Gruppen, L.D., Artino, A.R. Jr., Uijtdehaage, S., Szauter, K., and Durning, S.J. 2016. How to write an educational research grant: AMEE Guide No. 101. *Medical Teacher*, 38(2), 113–22. https://doi.org/10.3109/0142159X.2015.1087483

5. Gottlieb, M., Lee, S., Burkhardt, J., Carlson, J.N., King, A.M., Wong, A.H., and Santen, S.A. 2019. Show me the money: successfully obtaining grant

funding in medical education. *Western Journal of Emergency Medicine*, 20(1), 71. https://doi.org/10.5811/westjem.2018.10.41269

6. Cunningham, K. 2020. Beyond boundaries: developing grant writing skills across higher education institutions. *Journal of Research Administration*, 51(2), 41–57.

7. Ahn, H., and Reifsnider, E. 2021. A guide to writing grant proposals for nursing research. *Research in Nursing and Health*, 44(4), 596–7. https://doi.org/10.1002/nur.22137

8. Wiebe, N.G., and Maticka-Tyndale, E. 2017. More and better grant proposals? The evaluation of a grant-writing group at a mid-sized Canadian university. *Journal of Research Administration*, 48(2), 67–92.

9. Goff-Albritton, R.A., Cola, P.A., Pierre, J., Yerra, S.D., and Garcia, I. 2022. Faculty views on the barriers and facilitators to grant activities in the USA: a systematic literature review. *Journal of Research Administration*, 53(2), 14–39.

10. Cassell, H.M., Rose, E.S., Moon, T.D., Bello-Manga, H., Aliyu, M.H., and Mutale, W. 2022. Strengthening research capacity through an intensive training program for biomedical investigators from low-and middle-income countries: the Vanderbilt Institute for Research Development and Ethics (VIRDE). *BMC Medical Education*, 22(1), 1–3. https://doi.org/10.1186/s12909-022-03162-8

11. Weber-Main, A.M., Engler, J., McGee, R., Egger, M.J., Jones, H.P., Wood, C.V., Boman, K., Wu, J., Langi, A.K., and Okuyemi K.S. 2022. Variations of a group coaching intervention to support early-career biomedical researchers in grant proposal development: a pragmatic, four-arm, group-randomized trial. *BMC Medical Education*, 22(1), 1–6. https://doi.org/10.1186/s12909-021-03093-w

12. Guthrie, S., Rodriguez Rincon, D., McInroy, G., Ioppolo, B., and Gunashekar, S. 2019. Measuring bias, burden and conservatism in research funding processes. *F1000Research*, 8, 851. https://doi.org/10.12688/f1000research.19156.1

13. McDowell, G.S., Niziolek, C.A., and Lijek, R.S. 2021. How to bring peer review ghostwriters out of the dark. *Molecular Biology of the Cell*, 32(6), 461–6. https://doi.org/10.1091/mbc.E20-10-0642

14. Radder, H. 2023. How (not) to be held accountable in research: the case of the Dutch integrity code. *Accountability in Research*, 30(5), 261–75. https://doi.org/10.1080/08989621.2022.2115888

15. Dresler, M. 2022. FENS-Kavli Network of Excellence: postponed, non-competitive peer review for research funding. *European Journal of Neuroscience*, 58(12), 4441–8. https://doi.org/10.1111/ejn.15818

16. Dresler, M., Buddeberg, E., Endesfelder, U., Haaker, J., Hof, C., Kretschmer, R., Pflüger, D., and Schmidt, F. 2023. Effective or predatory

funding? Evaluating the hidden costs of grant applications. *Immunology and Cell Biology*, 101(2), 104–11. https://doi.org/10.1111/imcb.12592

17. Gopalakrishna, G., Wicherts, J.M., Vink, G., Stoop, I., van den Akker, O.R., Ter Riet, G., and Bouter, L.M. 2022. Prevalence of responsible research practices among academics in the Netherlands. *F1000Research*, 11, 471. https://doi.org/10.12688/f1000research.110664.2

18. Conix, S., De Block, A., and Vaesen, K. 2021. Grant writing and grant peer review as questionable research practices. *F1000Research*, 10, 1126. https://doi.org/10.12688/f1000research.73893.2

19. Eaton, L. 2005. Medical editors issue guidance on ghost writing. *BMJ*, 330(7498), 988. https://doi.org/10.1136/bmj.330.7498.988-a

20. Bosch, X. 2011. Treat ghostwriting as misconduct. *Nature*, 469(7331), 472. https://doi.org/10.1038/469472c

21. Artino, A.R. Jr., Driessen, E.W., and Maggio, L.A. 2019. Ethical shades of gray: international frequency of scientific misconduct and questionable research practices in health professions education. *Academic Medicine*, 94(1), 76–84. https://doi.org/10.1097/ACM.0000000000002412

22. Maggio, L.A., Artino, A.R. Jr., Watling, C.J., Driessen, E.W., and O'Brien, B.C. 2019. Exploring researchers' perspectives on authorship decision making. *Medical Education*, 53(12), 1253–62. https://doi.org/10.1111/medu.13950

23. McDowell, G.S., Knutsen, J.D., Graham, J.M., Oelker, S.K., and Lijek, R.S. 2019. Research culture: co-reviewing and ghostwriting by early-career researchers in the peer review of manuscripts. *Elife*, 8, e48425. https://doi.org/10.7554/eLife.48425

24. Maggio, L.A. 2021. Scholarly experiences in medical education: considering authorship. *Medical Education.*, 55(2), 138–9. https://doi.org/10.1111/medu.14417

25. Konopasky, A., O'Brien, B.C., Artino, A.R. Jr., Driessen, E.W., Watling, C.J., and Maggio, L.A. 2022. I, we and they: a linguistic and narrative exploration of the authorship process. *Medical Education*, 56(4), 456–64. https://doi.org/10.1111/medu.14697

26. Bourdieu, P. and Nice, R. 1980. The production of belief: contribution to an economy of symbolic goods. *Media, Culture and Society*, 2(3), 261–93. https://doi.org/10.1177/016344378000200305

27. Varpio, L., Albert M. 2013. AM last page: how Pierre Bourdieu's theory and concepts can apply to medical education. *Academic Medicine*, 88(8), 1189. https://doi.org/10.1097/ACM.0b013e31829d5815

28. Mendoza, P., Kuntz, A.M., and Berger, J.B. 2012. Bourdieu and academic capitalism: faculty "habitus" in materials science and engineering. *The Journal of Higher Education*, 83(4), 558–81. https://doi.org/10.1080/00221546.2012.11777257

29. Casad, B.J., Franks, J.E., Garasky, C.E., Kittleman, M.M., Roesler, A.C., Hall, D.Y., and Petzel, Z.W. 2021. Gender inequality in academia: problems and solutions for women faculty in STEM. *Journal of Neuroscience Research*, 99(1), 13–23. https://doi.org/10.1002/jnr.24631

30. Escobar, M., Bell, Z.K., Qazi, M., Kotoye, C.O., and Arcediano, F. 2021. Faculty time allocation at historically Black universities and its relationship to institutional expectations. *Frontiers in Psychology*, 4505. https://doi.org/10.3389/fpsyg.2021.734426

31. Hassouneh, D. 2017. *Faculty of Color in the Health Professions: Stories of Survival and Success*. Dartmouth College Press.

32. Franks, A.M., Calamur, N., Dobrian, A., Danielsen, M., Neumann, S.A., Cowan, E., and Weiler, T. 2022. Rank and tenure amongst faculty at academic medical centers: a study of more than 50 years of gender disparities. *Academic Medicine*, 97(7), 1038–48. https://doi.org/10.1097/ACM.0000000000004706

33. Bazeley, P., Kemp, L., Stevens, K., Asmar, C., Grbich, C., Marsh, H., and Bhathal, R. 1996. *Waiting in the Wings: A Study of Early Career Academic Researchers in Australia*. National Board of Employment, Education and Training, Australian Research Council. Available from: www.academia.edu/35549787/Waiting_in_the_Wings_A_Study_of_Early_Career_Academic_Researchers_in_Australia.

34. Lewiss, R.E., Silver, J.K., Bernstein, C.A., Mills, A.M., Overholser, B., and Spector, N.D. 2020. Is academic medicine making mid-career women physicians invisible? *Journal of Women's Health*, 29(2), 187–92. https://doi.org/10.1089/jwh.2019.7732

35. Cavanagh, A., Jabbar, A., and Vanstone, M. 2021. Particularising "experiences": naming whiteness in the academy. *Medical Education*, 55(5), 548–50. https://doi.org/10.1111/medu.14451

36. Varpio, L., Harvey, E., Jaarsma, D., Dudek, N., Hay, M., Day, K., Bader Larsen, K., and Cleland, J. 2021. Attaining full professor: women's and men's experiences in medical education. *Medical Education*, 55(5), 582–94. https://doi.org/10.1111/medu.14392

37. Kleinfelder, J., Price, J.H., and Dake, J.A. 2003. Grant writing: practice and preparation of university health educators. *American Journal of Health Education*, 34(1), 47–53. https://doi.org/10.1080/19325037.2003.10603525

38. Russo, E. 2003. Victims of success. *Nature*, 422(6929), 354–5. Available from: https://link.gale.com/apps/doc/A187661638/HRCA?u=anon~7fe47979&sid=googleScholar&xid=0f884fa7

39. Kennedy, D., Austin, J., Urquhart, K., and Taylor, C. 2004. Supply without demand. *Science*, 303(5661), 1105. https://doi.org/10.1126/science.303.5661.1105

40. Zierler, B.K., Summerside, N., Sprecher, J., Blakeney, E., Vogel, M., Chu, F., and Posner, J.D. 2021. 16506 Recognizing interdisciplinary collaborative

research in promotion and tenure processes. *Journal of Clinical and Translational Science*, 5(s1), 110. https://doi.org/10.1017/cts.2021.681

41. Anderson, M.S., Horn, A.S., Risbey, K.R., Ronning, E.A., De Vries, R., and Martinson, B.C. 2007. What do mentoring and training in the responsible conduct of research have to do with scientists' misbehavior? Findings from a National Survey of NIH-funded scientists. Academic Medicine, 82(9), 853–60. https://doi.org/10.1097/ACM.0b013e31812f764c

42. Anderson, M.S., Ronning, E.A., De Vries, R., and Martinson, B.C. 2007. The perverse effects of competition on scientists' work and relationships. *Science and Engineering Ethics*, 13, 437–61. https://doi.org/10.1007/s11948-007-9042-5

43. Reardon, S. 2021. "We're problem solvers": research administrators offer guidance to working scientists. *Nature*, 595(7866), 321–2. https://doi.org/10.1038/d41586-021-01829-8

44. Whitchurch, C. 2012. *Reconstructing Identities in Higher Education: The Rise of Third Space Professionals*. Routledge.

45. Coaldrake, P., and Stedman, L. 1999. *Academic Work in the Twenty-First Century*. Higher Education Division, Training and Youth Affairs, Canberra.

46. Zink, H.R., Hughes, D., and Vanderford, N.L. 2022. Reconfiguring the research administration workforce: a qualitative study explaining the increasingly diverse professional roles in research administration. *Journal of Research Administration*, 53(2).

47. Barnett, R. 2000. *Realizing the University in an Age of Supercomplexity*. McGraw-Hill Education.

48. Mosier, K.E. 2022. Deconstructing the art of grantsmanship: the roles of the storyteller, grant writer, typesetter, proofreader, accountant and reviewer. *Journal of Research Administration*, 53(1), 93–121.

49. Lunt, I. 2008. Ethical issues in professional life. In *Exploring Professionalism*, edited by B. Cunningham, 88–98. Bedford Way Papers.

50. Smith, C., Holden, M., Yu, E., and Hanlon, P. 2021. "So what do you do?": third space professionals navigating a Canadian university context. *Journal of Higher Education Policy and Management*, 43(5), 505–19. https://doi.org/10.1080/1360080X.2021.1884513

51. Carter-Edwards, L., Grewe, M.E., Fair, A.M., Jenkins, C., Ray, N.J., Bilheimer, A., Dave, G., et al. 2021. Recognizing cross-institutional fiscal and administrative barriers and facilitators to conducting community-engaged clinical and translational research. *Academic Medicine*, 96(4), 558. https://doi.org/10.1097/ACM.0000000000003893

52. Musselin, C. 2007. *The Transformation of Academic Work: Facts and Analysis*. Research and Occasional Paper Series: CSHE 4.07. Center for Studies in Higher Education.

Institutional Concerns

15 Institutional Concerns – Framing Chapter: The Invisible People and Processes That Bring Life to Our Education Institutions

JONATHAN SHERBINO

The world is full of magic things, patiently waiting for our senses to grow sharper.

– W.B. Yeats.

I began my academic life as a clinical trialist. And after a short but spectacular failure, I revived my academic aspirations when I discovered the field of health professions education (HPE). Entering graduate school in higher education, specifically HPE, I was lost. The language, the literature, the assumptions, the paradigms, and more were unfamiliar. Yet, they were source material for a curiosity that energized me. In time, I developed a community of teachers, mentors, and peers that helped me learn the code, provide new ways of seeing, push back unconscious assumptions, and guide me as I waded into the HPE literature. My graduate school thesis was the evaluation of a novel teaching framework for the "unique" teaching environment of the emergency department. My first addition to the HPE literature addressed the dyad of teacher and learner.

The teacher-learner dyad is a key focus of the HPE literature. Until I was asked to write this chapter, I missed a gap in the literature. In hindsight, I now see it is a large gap. Teaching and learning in the health professions is dominated by attention to either the student or teacher. Absent are the many other essential people who make education possible. The community that launched me as a clinician educator, and which supports me today, is invisible in the literature and absent from the conversations in the field. If you are sceptical of this claim, conduct a quick literature search. Search HPE plus administrator or technology support. There will be no (well, almost no) relevant returns. While reflecting on this gap, I'm keenly aware that my graduate school experience was made possible by a multitude of dedicated people. My training was enabled by the administrators, technologists, accreditors, faculty developers, and others who maintained an effective and functioning program, complete with resources to support learning, and who achieved an educational standard that was consistently delivered by up-to-date teachers. How quickly did my initial foray into HPE research narrow the learning environment to a function of only student and teacher. The infrastructure necessary to support my learning and my research was neither appreciated nor articulated.

This book, and specifically this third section, brings attention to all the institutional players that make the learning environment – and hence learning – possible. The goal is to help sharpen our senses, to make the invisible visible, and to rediscover the "magic" that brings life to our education institutions. I have considered the appropriate metaphor to bring a fresh perspective to the interconnectedness of the institution – teaching hospital, ambulatory clinic, academic department, university – and have passed on the tired metaphors of an orchestra or sports team. Except for the conductor or coach, the musicians and players look very much alike. Rather, and appropriate for the health professions, an educational institution is like a living cell. A cell contains various organelles – nucleus, endoplasmic reticulum, ribosomes, Golgi bodies, and more – each playing a unique role that is essential for the functioning of a cell. An organelle does not exist outside of a cell. A cell does not function without the interplay of processes necessary for life, such as reproduction, energy generation, protein synthesis, and protein transportation as provided by the organelles. And (without getting into the debate of viruses and prions) only organelles working together to accomplish their processes make life possible.

My point is that without the blueprints for courses of instruction, the learning technologies that facilitate search and communication, the maintenance of education standards, the continuing development of teacher competence, and more, the dyadic interplay between teacher and learner would rapidly degrade; the long and complex journey we have all taken in our learning careers – from primary school, to undergraduate education, to professional or graduate training – simply could not happen. Educating a healthcare provider doesn't happen in an ad hoc, serendipitous manner. It is deeply organized and interconnected. All the parts of that educational trajectory are reliant on each other. Like the cell, it works because all the parts are present and functioning.

Indeed, while this section of this book is entitled *Institutional Concerns*, an institution is not a building. The COVID-19 pandemic taught us that our education practices can (with varying success) move to virtual environments. Certainly, we must acknowledge the fiscal and technological barriers to virtual environments in some jurisdictions, particularly the Global South. And of course, HPE is a special case of higher education, in part because of the unique requirement of clinical education (i.e., "bedside" teaching), which is not currently transferable into the virtual environment (until augmented or virtual reality technologies make significant gains). Nonetheless, it is not classrooms, lecture halls, and offices that make an institution; rather, it is the people and processes. And it is the process and the people that bring education to life.

Collaborative processes and teams of people bring to mind Peter Senge's concept of a learning organization, which is defined as a context "where people continually expand their capacity to create the results they truly desire, where new and expansive patterns of thinking are nurtured, where collective aspiration is set free, and where people are continually learning to see the whole together."[1 (p.3)] Perhaps Senge intentionally omitted the term "institution" from this description because it carries a tacit reference to bureaucracy, lack of creativity, risk-avoidance, and more. None of these connotations are part of Senge's learning organization. In contrast, a learning organization adopts processes that empower people to advance the mission of the organization personally and collectively. Our best version of HPE institutions reflect the characteristics of learning organizations.

People in learning organizations are committed to ongoing learning and development, desiring to grow professionally and make significant contributions in their roles. However, learning in isolation is less impactful than team learning, where networks are emphasized, allowing collective needs to inform learning and facilitate rapid sharing of ideas and solutions. In learning organizations, processes include systems thinking; complexity is considered by looking at the whole of the problem and evaluating relationships rather than applying reductionistic strategies that impair sensemaking. In learning organizations, the fidelity of information is corrupted as parts of the whole lose relational connectedness. Systems thinking is reinforced via the use of shared mental models, so that assumptions, priorities, and goals are common across people. And finally, a learning organization has a shared vision.[1]

Examining the education of health professionals through the lens of learning organizations highlights a contradiction that can stymie HPE: integrating the systems thinking of learning organizations is challenged by our field's focus on learning, teaching, and performing at an individual level. While an individual may feel accountability to the goals of the institution, the individual often lacks the formal power to change the necessary policies when they obstruct the achievement of that goal. Argyris argues that human action is a consequence of design. Learning organizations can address the issue of power that suppresses interdependent collaboration via intentional advocacy that inquires about others' views with follow-up testing of new ideas.[2] Together, "Senge's approach engages participants in substantive strategic issues, while Argyris helps them to develop critical reasoning and communication skills for learning."[3] [(p. 17)] Framed this way, our education institutions should seek to value all the (invisible) people engaged in the education enterprise, using processes that can address the complexity necessary to serve HPE. Health professional education should never reduce to the simplistic (tokenistic?) dyad of teacher and student.

In this section of *A Chorus of Unheard Voices*, authors bring into perspective the institutional infrastructure necessary for HPE. Connected via the metaphor of the cell, a summary of the invisible people and processes that inform education institutions is discussed below.

People

The people of HPE institutions include, among others, technicians, administrators, and faculty developers. In Chapter 17 technology professionals are seen, I suspect, for the first time in the HPE literature. Technology professionals support the energy system (i.e., mitochondria) of our education institutions. They include audio-visual specialists, computer network specialists, learning management system experts, and instructional designers, among others. Without these professionals to build, support, and troubleshoot the technologies that provide the platforms for learning, our institutions fail. (WiFi has been suggested to be either the pinnacle or the base of Maslow's hierarchy of needs, depending on your perspective.) In the absence of technology, contemporary education would be severely limited and even not possible in many institutions, particularly in centres using a distributed education model.

This chapter on technology professionals examines their role in procurement, deployment, design, and maintenance of various technologies. Sociomaterialism provides a construct to examine the intersection of technology and learning.[4] Technology is not neutral to human interaction and behaviour. The selection and implementation of technology will both facilitate and inhibit learning in various (and often unpredictable) ways. Effective educators partner with technology professionals to understand the implications of material objects, technologies, and infrastructure on their teaching. This chapter brings the concept of sociomaterialism to life via the lived experience of various technicians.

Chapter 18 turns our attention to the crucial work completed by HPE's administrative staff members. The progressive, global transition of HPE to a competency-based education model requires sophisticated systems to accommodate sequenced progression of training and tailored learning experiences.[5] Further, programmatic assessment generates data and requires systems to aggregate and present these data in a reliable and meaningful way. This increasing sophistication of education design requires administrative coordination and oversight. This chapter is a case study of postgraduate medical education administration, examining the clerical, managerial, and learner support roles of program administration coordinators (PACs). The case study compares training backgrounds and responsibilities between North America and Europe. Continuing the cell metaphor, PACs are the cytoskeleton. Too frequently unseen by the institution, although frequently acknowledged by learners and clinician educators, the PAC ensures the structure and stability of an education program.

Next, Chapter 20 highlights the vital role played by faculty developers. Defining faculty development is challenging, an example of how the absence of a lingua franca in HPE muddies the literature. Depending on local context, faculty development might represent academic development, professional development, or teacher training. Faculty development refers to all activities that health professionals pursue to improve their knowledge, skills, and behaviours as clinicians, educators, leaders, and scholars, in both individual and group settings.[6] In this chapter, the faculty developer is introduced as mediating the complex, liminal space between institutional imperatives and the individual's needs and career goals. This service of institutional and individual needs requires the synthesis and delivery of educational resources (e.g., the function of the endoplasmic reticulum). The term "development" speaks to growth, but it can also suggest insufficient achievement, positioning the faculty developer in potential conflict when established professionals are required to attend an initiative aimed at their "development."

Processes

In parallel with (invisible) people that make HPE institutions possible are (invisible) processes. Chapter 19 examines the accreditation process, which evaluates the quality of education programs against defined standards to ensure quality and promote continuous improvement. Accreditation's magic lies in the thoughtful dialogue between expert reviewers and the constituents (e.g., teachers, learners, administrators) of a program. When done well, accreditation validates the investments and creativity of a program and provides insights into areas of future development. When done poorly, accreditation can devolve into bureaucratic paperwork. Visiting accreditors (who audit and report on an institution and associated programs), institutional champions (who coordinate internal and external reviews), and program directors (who complete self-studies of their programs), are unseen by the education institution, yet the success of programs, and the accreditation enterprise overall, depends on their work. The accreditation process is much like the transcription of DNA into RNA within the nucleus, ensuring the code of the cell is made available for the subsequent translation of RNA into a protein. Accreditation stimulates changes to the curriculum and learning environment, protects trainees from bad training, and shields the public from unprepared graduates.

In Chapter 21, the risks for learners inherent in HPE, including psychological distress, mental illness, and identity dissonance, is examined. Supporting the well-being of future clinicians requires a collective process, one that cannot be delegated to a specific person and then ignored. Via the narrative of a student affairs dean and a clinical psychologist, a central argument is made that supporting the well-being of health professional learners requires both holistic support of individuals and environmental reform. To combat high rates of depression, burnout, and anxiety, interventions such as duty hour limitations, stress management training, support group meetings, mindfulness interventions, and curricular reform have been made. However, these interventions have had limited impact on learner well-being. This inconsistent effect raises concerns about a collective understanding of what it means to be well or unwell while engaged in HPE. Focusing on solving learner impairment without addressing its underlying systemic causes may further entrench impaired well-being and miss opportunities for resilience development. Much like the lysosome of a cell, which targets intracellular debris that impairs cellular function, the process of supporting learner well-being is a clinical and moral imperative for education institutions.

Finally, Chapter 16 speaks to the renewal of our institutions by redressing the inequity of a medical profession only available to young, white, cisgender, heterosexual, and male physicians. The process of ensuring justice, equity, diversity, and inclusion often reduces to a singular focus by institutions on diversity, leaving the responsibility of equity and inclusion to students who remain invisible to the institution. Through the voice of a first-generation, low-income medical student, we hear how our HPE institutions must work to create equitable and inclusive environments. The plasma membrane of a cell maintains the balance of factors necessary for life. In the absence of energy to support cell membrane transporters, homeostasis is lost. The active process of seeking equity, diversity, and inclusiveness in our institutions is essential for the life of HPE.

Concluding Thoughts

An institution is formed by the interplay of the people and processes that make its mission possible. While the architectural brutalism of buildings preferred by health and education systems cannot be unseen, it is easy to miss the people and processes of HPE institutions who are outside of the teacher and learner roles. This section seeks to help "our senses to grow sharper" and make visible essential elements of our institutions largely ignored in the literature. In the absence of people – technology professionals, administrators, faculty developers – and processes – accreditation; supporting well-being; creating equitable, diverse, and inclusive institutions – health professions education is impossible.

References

1. Senge, P.M. 2006. *The Fifth Discipline: The Art and Practice of the Learning Organization*. Doubleday.
2. Argyris, C. 1993. *Actionable Knowledge: Changing the Status Quo*. Jossey-Bass.
3. Edmondson, A., and Moingeon, B. 1998. From organizational learning to the learning organization. *Management Learning*, 29(1), 5–20. https://doi.org/10.1177/1350507698291001
4. Burm, S., and MacLeod, A. 2020. A sense of sociomaterialism: how sociomaterial perspectives might illuminate health professions education. *Focus on Health Professional Education: A Multi-disciplinary Journal*, 21(1), 1–2. https://doi.org/10.11157/fohpe.v21i1.443
5. Van Melle, E., Frank, J.R., Holmboe, E.S., Dagnone, D., Stockley, D., and Sherbino, J. 2019. A core components framework for evaluating implementation of competency-based medical education programs. *Academic Medicine*, 94(7), 1002–9. https://doi.org/10.1097/ACM.0000000000002743
6. Steinert, Y. 2020. Faculty development: from rubies to oak. *Medical Teacher*, 42(4), 429–35. https://doi.org/10.1080/0142159X.2019.1688769

16 "On the Backs of Students": Addressing Diversity, Equity, Inclusion, and Accessibility in Medical Education

TASHA R. WYATT, BASSEL SHANAB, AND GARETH GINGELL

Even to this day, it only takes one accident. My scholarship does not only pay for my livelihood, it covers that of my entire family. I fail out? There goes rent; there goes the tuition money for my siblings' education; then, the cars are sold off and job prospects limited to accessible transportation options. It'd be just a matter of time before the circle completed itself. All four of my family members living in a squalid basement, with dreams and aspirations of a better life

– Bassel Shanab, medical student

Across the Global North, medical schools are prioritizing diversity, equity, inclusion (DEI), and accessibility in medical education. This move challenges the historical precedent that the profession is only available to physicians who are young, white, able, cisgender, heterosexual, and male, and that medical training should centre around their needs.[1] In the last few years, much work has been done to address some of the problematic underlying architecture that has made medical education exclusive to this population, including challenging issues related to racism,[2] sexism,[3] and ableism.[4] However, while many medical schools have formalized DEI positions to address these issues, medical students continue to be heavily invested, engaging in this invisible work despite not being credited.[5]

Students are often at the forefront of DEI work. They use their experiences as marginalized people, immigrants, gender minorities, racial minorities, etc. to identify problems and seek change. They display ongoing acts of resistance by raising questions about the reasons that underlie the design of medical schools, by addressing curricular materials that negatively position already socially marginalized groups, and by engaging in marches, protests, and boycotts as means to challenge the status quo. However, because of their subject position within the

hierarchy of medicine, students' acts are frequently rendered invisible –
overlooked by leadership or viewed as mere annoyances rather than as
the actions of change agents within a system that was not designed for
learners like them.

In this chapter, as two medical education researchers, we explore
the invisible work of one medical student, Bassel, taking on an often-
invisible topic in medical education – *medical student food insecurity*.
Limited access to food is related to individuals' socioeconomic status
(SES), which is not given the same level of attention in medical school
as other issues of identity, such as race and gender. Rather, by virtue
of pursuing medicine as a profession, it is assumed that students have
the financial and social resources needed to successfully navigate and
participate in the system.[6–8] However, low SES, food insecurity, and
classism greatly affects medical students' training in terms of their
ability to concentrate, perform, and succeed in medical school.[9–11] Further, this particular student's identity is highly intersectional, and his
experiences as a Muslim Palestinian American born to a single mother
of three children give him a unique perspective on DEI work. At the
cross-section of being an immigrant suffering from financial instability within a traditionally economically and socially privileged space,
he occupies an often-overlooked space in medical education. His story
lends insight into how students' basic needs of food and shelter can
easily go unmet, and how students' lived experiences with these unmet
needs can reshape DEI work in impactful ways.

History of Equity, Diversity, and Inclusion in the USA and Academic Medicine

As a result of the protests and civil action of the 1960s, military, business, and educational institutions across the USA began to focus on
issues of racial diversity.[12] This deepened the awareness around racial
inequality that swept through the country during the Civil Rights
movement alongside increasing anti-discriminatory legislation and a
growing sensitivity to issues of social justice.[13] However, the value of
having a diverse workforce was realized much later. It was not until
the 1990s and 2000s, with now decades of data on racial diversity in the
workplace, that researchers could report on the positive outcomes of
diversity for corporations, such as greater employee retention, workforce problem-solving ability, and workplace engagement.

However, while corporations and institutions of higher education
have begun to realize the importance of diversity in reaching their
goals, medical schools and the healthcare workforce have lagged

behind.[14] At present, most medical schools report the importance of having a racially diverse student body, but other kinds of diversity, such as the unique experiences of first-generation college students[15] have only recently been noticed. These oversights exist because leaders make assumptions about their learners' homogeneity, overlooking that most student populations vary immensely by race, ethnicity, SES, and age.[16] In a system where those in positions of power and authority fail to anticipate the needs of a diverse population of learners, what often results is that the struggles faced by individuals go unaddressed until students raise an institution's awareness. In other words, while institutions have focused on issues of diversity in DEI work, the responsibility of equity and inclusion are frequently left to students. Through their campaigns to raise awareness, students educate their leaders on what should be done to create equitable and inclusive environments.[5]

Research shows first-generation and low-income (FGLI) students face multiple challenges that prevent them from easily manoeuvring in the academic system,[17–19] including financial instability, access to professional networks, and behavioural scripts for how to project oneself as a physician. Many tend to be older students with commitments to their immediate and extended families.[20] They are often children of immigrants or are immigrants themselves, and a significant number are also underrepresented in medicine (UIM).[21] Additionally, many are from low-income backgrounds with a household annual income under US$25,000,[20] which subjects them and their families to ongoing housing and food insecurity.

Despite the efforts of the American Association for Medical Colleges (AAMC) to address the challenges these students experience,[22] this diverse population continues to report unique needs that are unmet by their institutions, which have fallen short of addressing equity and inclusion. As such, FGLI students are engaged in invisible DEI work in an attempt to raise awareness around the kinds of support they need to succeed as medical trainees. As Bassel explains, these students are key to identifying aspects of the institutional system that fail to work for various groups of students, a reality that frequently falls below the radar.

Bassel's Invisible Work

In Bassel's work to raise the issue of food insecurity among the FGLI population, he draws upon the idea that the USA is imbued with oppressive structures. In Bassel's words, which echo those of others,[23] "America is a complicated country with a history, to this present day, of dominating people via physical and financial means." As a FGLI student, he has struggled on multiple levels as he works to finish his educational training. During high school, for example, he lived in a one-bedroom apartment with his mother and two siblings. Not only did they struggle to pay their rent, but they also had to hide the number of people living in the apartment. Because Bassel was not on the lease, he could not receive mail with his name on it, which prevented college flyers from reaching him. He received meals from his school's free lunch program during this time. He did not fully realize the limitations of this program until he tried to select something different in the cafeteria line than what he had always chosen. As he explains,

It wasn't until I tried to select a deli sandwich with a side of fruit that I was told I would have to pay. I had been receiving free lunch for a long time. Class field trips were covered or fees for some type of school event were covered, but it was only then did I realize just what that looked like.

Bassel's struggle with food insecurity intensified in college where, as a pre-medical student, he would take a shuttle to Chicago to work in an off-campus lab at his college's affiliated medical school for 20 hours a week. He had early wake times and long afternoons, which prevented him from accessing the dining hall where his meal plan paid for his meals.

I would often take the last campus shuttle out of Chicago, arriving after the dining halls closed down. With no money to waste on vending machines, I'd subsist on anything I could find, from candy/snacks to (unfortunately) theft from vending machines. I was ashamed of what I had done, but I was not eating. I had called the University's Dining Services to explain to them what I was facing. There were no dining halls nor options those first few months, and I was starving for nights at a time. I remember not being able to focus, just drinking water in an attempt to quench my hunger.

This experience of food insecurity affected all areas of his life, and the struggles poured into his personal life. As a pre-medical student, he had all the "traditional" marks of being successful, including good grades and leadership positions. But, as he explained, "I was suffering from food insecurity and imposter syndrome at what I thought was my big break. I thought I left it all behind me, the forever oppressive poverty." However, his struggle with food insecurity persisted into medical education. Training for an elite profession was not enough to save him from these circumstances.

Further, the varied array of privileged and oppressed identities intersecting in the FGLI population (i.e., race, gender, immigration status,

SES) make it complicated to raise issues around their needs, particularly if they are viewed as a homogeneous group. Bassel's description demonstrates the complexity of these students: "I am not just a low-income student at a primarily white institution. I am a Muslim Palestinian American. I am a first-born son to a conservative Middle Eastern single mother of three children." Knowing this particular intersection of identities was not universal, Bassel was keenly aware that, in college, if he drew attention to his particular struggles, he might unintentionally draw attention away from others' needs. This left him conflicted about his role in DEI work, "It felt selfish to advocate [for those who fit this category] when other student voices are also rightfully calling for attention to campus police brutality and perpetuations of racism." He was aware that there were "resources meant to help marginalized students," but because he was not from a well-recognized group, any attempts at raising awareness could be detrimental to his peers, "I was not a Black or Hispanic student; I did not feel like I should consume such hard-fought resources."

However, his experiences with food insecurity in medical school marked what he describes as "a series of maturation and burgeoning responsibilities." As he struggled for food in a system that "doesn't support all students," he gained confidence in approaching leadership about his specific struggles. His account of his unabated food insecurity finally reached senior administrators at the Yale School of Medicine, who approached him to assist with the creation of a grocery store survey. The survey asked preclinical students "what [they] were buying (take-out, meal prep ingredients) from where (stores' locations) and how (delivery subscriptions, carpools)" to map how they were interacting with food. Following this, he was invited by various deans to continue a research project on food insecurity as a way to provide evidence that this was indeed a problem at this elite institution. Recognizing that his issues were finally getting attention, he accepted formal roles to work on behalf of the institutions' DEI efforts. As he says, "I aspire to change the system. To allow for an overhaul of process and policy for such systemic underserving of marginalized populations." Guiding his work in DEI is his own experience in having "critical unmet needs," and using these experiences to work on behalf of others "to advocate for change." Change, however, cannot happen if voices and experiences are not heard and remain unknown.

Concluding Thoughts

From Bassel's perspective, although working towards DEI is critical in medical education, institutions have shirked their responsibility and left students to address equity and inclusion. This is further exacerbated when they are taught about the social determinants of health, including patients' experiences of housing instability, transportation, and insurance access. Typically, they learn from clinicians who espouse dominant historical perspectives and signal that such work is "social work" and *not* the responsibility of physicians. These kinds of messages leave students wondering what role medical institutions play in doing DEI work other than acknowledging the importance of diversity and that patients experience challenges. These messages also decontextualize patients from their social environment and the factors that contribute to their poor health.

This invisible work is left largely to students who already have marginalized identities and themselves struggle within the system. When we asked Bassel why he does the invisible work of DEI at his medical school, his answer points to a system not made for him or his peers. He wants senior administrators to be honest about this situation: "We have always had students of color, students of FGLI, students of minority gender and sex, etc. doing the teaching for classmates struggling to comprehend patient barriers." Even though his efforts often go unrecognized, it is critical for moving the profession forward and ensuring the humane treatment of patients. Students must do this work because medical schools have not seen this as their responsibility, thus leaving students with no choice.

Clinically, attending to students' unmet needs are critical for them "to become successful enough to become providers." When students are unable to have enough food to sustain their gruelling schedule or enough money to afford housing on away rotations, it becomes challenging to do much of anything else but merely survive. Therefore, students like Bassel fight to reframe how the system views medical students – not as a universally wealthy and privileged group, but as the diverse, and potentially vulnerable, population that they are. If they cannot meet their needs in medical school, the chances are that they might not graduate to do the work necessary as a practising physician. From Bassel's perspective, he does this work to ensure his classmates make it to the finish line so that they can actually become physicians: "DEI work gives those latter students a fighting chance by sufficiently providing for them as they attempt the next step in academic medicine."

Additional Reading

Flynn, M., Monteiro, K., George, P., Tunkel, A. 2020. Assessing food insecurity in medical students. *Family Medicine*, 52(7), 512–3. https://doi.org/10.22454/fammed.2020.722238

Thorman, A. and Dhillon, H. 2021. No food for thought: document-ing the prevalence of food insecurity among medical students at one Western university. *Journal of Hunger & Environmental Nutrition*, 16(5), 643–9. https://doi.org/10.1080/19320248.2021.1873885

Smith, S., Malinak, D., Chang, J., Schultz, A., and Brownwell, K. 2017. Addressing food insecurity in family medicine and medical education. *Family Medicine*, 49(10), 765–71. PMID: 29190401. https://pubmed.ncbi.nlm.nih.gov/29190401/

Disclaimer: This work was prepared by a civilian employee of the U.S. Government as part of the individual's official duties and therefore is in the public domain. The opinions and assertions expressed herein are those of the author(s) and do not necessarily reflect the official policy or position of the Uniformed Services University or the Department of Defense.

References

1. LeBlanc, C., Sonnenberg, L., King, S., and Busari, J. 2020. Medical educa-tion leadership: from diversity to inclusivity. *GMS Journal for Medical Education*, 37(2), Doc18. https://doi.org/10.3205/zma001311

2. Taiko, M., South, E., and Ray, V. 2021. Medical schools as racialized organi-zations: a primer. *Annals of Internal Medicine*, 174(8), 1143–4. https://doi.org/10.7326/M21-0369

3. Blalock, E., and Leal, D. 2022. Redressing injustices: how women students enact agency in undergraduate medical education. *Advances in Health Sci-ences Education*, 28, 741–58. https://doi.org/10.1007/s10459-022-10183-x

4. Jain, N. 2020. Political disclosure: resisting ableism in medical education. *Disability & Society*, 35(3), 389–412. https://doi.org/10.1080/09687599.2019.1647149

5. Moss, J., Hardy, E., Cooley, K., Cuffe, M., Lang, M., and Kennedy, A. 2020. Students advocating for diversity in medical education [version 2]. *MedEd-Publish*, 8, 159. https://doi.org/10.15694/mep.2019.000159.2

6. Beagan, B., MacLeod, A., Owen, M., Pride, T., and Sibbald, K. 2022. Lower-class origin professionals in Canadian health and social service profes-sions: "a different level of understanding". *Social Science & Medicine*, 309, 115233. https://doi.org/10.1016/j.socscimed.2022.115233

7. Beagan, B. 2005. Everyday classism in medical school: experiencing mar-ginality and resistance. *Medical Education*, 39(8), 777–84. https://doi.org/10.1111/j.1365-2929.2005.02225.x

8. Beagan, B. 2001. Micro inequities and everyday inequalities: "race", gender, sexuality and class in medical school. *Canadian Journal of Sociology*, 26(4), 583–610. https://doi.org/10.2307/3341493

9. Flynn, M., Monteiro, K., George, P., and Tunkel, A. 2020. Assessing food insecurity in medical students. *Family Medicine*, 52(7), 512–3. https://doi.org/10.22454/FamMed.2020.722238

10. Thorman, A., and Dhillon, H. 2021. No food for thought: documenting the prevalence of food insecurity among medical students at one Western university. *Journal of Hunger and Environmental Nutrition*, 16(5), 643–9. https://doi.org/10.1080/19320248.2021.1873885

11. Smith, S., Malinak, D., Chang, J., Schultz, A., and Brownwell, K. 2017. Addressing food insecurity in family medicine and medical education. *Family Medicine*, 49(10), 765–71.

12. Vaughn, B. 2007. The history of diversity training and its pioneers. *Strategic Diversity and Inclusion Management Magazine*, 1(1), 11–16. Available from: https://diversityofficermagazine.com/diversity-inclusion/the-history-of-diversity-training-its-pioneers/

13. Rosenkranz, K., Arora, T., Termuhlen P, Stain, S.C., Misra, S., Dent, D., and Nfonsam, V. 2021. Diversity, equity and inclusion in medicine: why it matters and how do we achieve it? *Journal of Surgical Education*, 78(4), 1058–65. https://doi.org/10.1016/j.jsurg.2020.11.013

14. Association of American Medical Colleges. nd. Addressing and eliminating racism at the AAMC and beyond. Accessed October 7, 2020. Available from: www.aamc.org/addressing-and-eliminating-racism-aamc-and-beyond.

15. Mason, H., Ata, A., Nguyen M, Nakae, S., Chakraverty, D., Eggan, B., Martinez, S., and Jeffe, D.B. 2022. First-generation and continuing-generation college graduates' application, acceptance, and matriculation to US medical schools: a national cohort study. *Medical Education Online*, 27(1), 1–11. https://doi.org/10.1080/10872981.2021.2010291

16. Hendrickson, R., Lane, J., Harris, J., and Borman, R. 2013. *Academic Leadership and Governance of Higher Education: A Guide for Trustees, Leaders, and Aspiring Leaders of Two- And Four-Year Institutions*. Stylus.

17. Colturi, J. 2021. "We are the underdogs": first-gen physicians on their pursuit of a medical career. *Op-Med*, November 16. Accessed May 1, 2022. Available from: https://opmed.doximity.com/articles/we-are-the-underdogs-first-gen-physicians-on-their-pursuit-of-a-medical-career?.

18. Sims, L. 2022. Into the unknown: experiences of social newcomers entering medical education. *Academic Medicine*, 97(10), 1528–35. https://doi.org/10.1097/ACM.0000000000004762

19. Yosso, T.J. 2005. Whose culture has capital? *Race, Ethnicity, and Education*, 8(1), 69–91. https://doi.org/10.1080/1361332052000341006

20. Engle, J., and Tinto, V. 2008. *Moving Beyond Access: College Success for Low-Income, First-Generation Students*. The Pell Institute. Available from: https://files.eric.ed.gov/fulltext/ED504448.pdf

21. Adachi, F. 1979. *Analysis of the First-Generation College Student Population: A New Concept in Higher Education*. University of Wyoming Division of Student Educational Opportunity.

22. Association of American Medical Colleges. nd. Tools and resources for first-generation medical school students. Accessed April 1, 2022. Available from: www.aamc.org/professional-development/affinity-groups/gea/first-generation-students.

23. DuBois, W.E.B. 1903/1989. *The Souls of Black Folks*. Chicago, IL: A. C. McClurg and Co.

17 The Invisible Work of Technology Professionals

ANITA SAMUEL, JASON WEINER, MICHAEL J. BATTISTONE, ANDREA M. BARKER, AND ERIN BARRY

There's been a tremendous evolution in how we use technology in medical education. It needs a specialized skill set to work with the different technologies. Especially because we're talking of interconnected systems that are at play, it's not just the audio-visual equipment or the PowerPoint slides. It's all of them working together. So, for a faculty member to teach, they need to know how the PowerPoint software works and create a slide deck that is visually appealing and reduces cognitive load. Faculty need to be able to use the audio-visual equipment in various classrooms and understand how institutional learning management platforms operate. Institutions have technology professionals specifically for audio-visual equipment or learning management systems. It's not feasible to expect one person to have expertise in all of these areas, yet that is what is being asked of faculty. We need to recognize that faculty can be far more effective in teaching their subject matter if they have support. Technology professionals working in tandem with faculty can help to create effective learning experiences for learners.

– Anita Samuel, Associate Professor and Associate
Director of Distance Learning

What is technology in medical education? Let's take the example of a medical school lecture to see the interplay of technologies and technology professionals.

Traditional lectures are delivered in classrooms equipped with, at a minimum, projectors, microphones, speakers, cameras, and a computer for the visual presentation. Most educators know the audio-visual (AV) professionals who maintain and troubleshoot this equipment. However, technology support for a lecture starts far ahead of the lecture. Technology professionals evaluate the presentation software and hardware based on their features, the privacy policies and implications for students and faculty, and cost implications for the organization before procurement. Technology professionals deploy and maintain

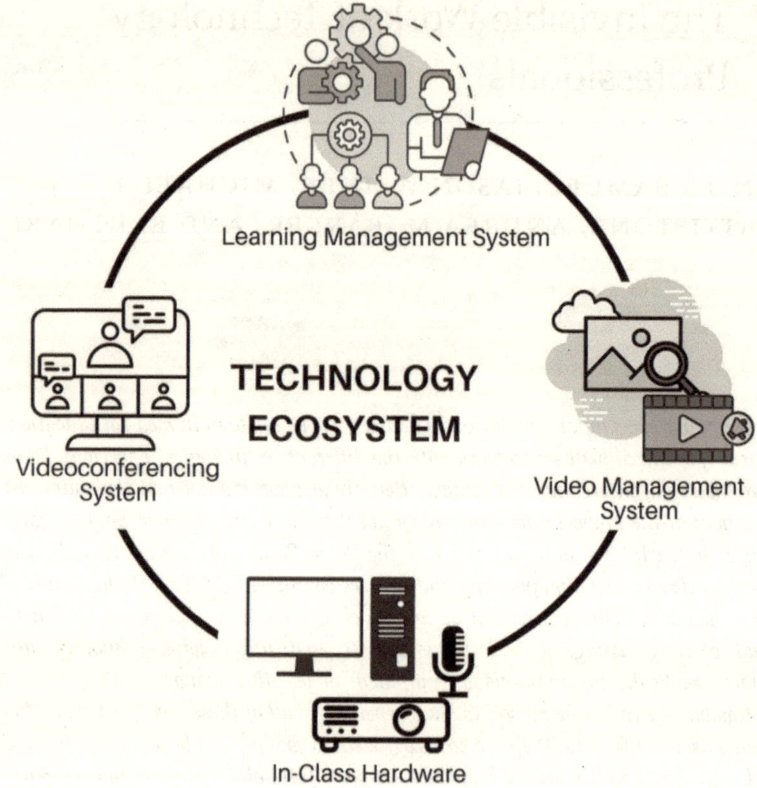

Figure 17.1 Higher education instructional technology ecosystem

the software and hardware across the organization upon procurement and simultaneously provide faculty training and support. Before the lecture, there may be pre-work assigned to learners that needs to be loaded into the learning management system (LMS) that other technology professionals may manage. As Erin summarizes, "giving a lecture" is a phrase that obscures a lot of work:

> *It's not just giving a lecture – so much goes into preparing materials for the lecture and hosting that session. Not everyone attending the session – even those involved in the teaching – appreciate all the work that makes it happen.*
> – Erin Barry, technology professional and assistant professor

Technology is deeply integrated into education, and educators work within a technology ecosystem. This ecosystem comprises a collection

Table 17.1 Technology professionals' job descriptions

Audio-visual professional	Set up and run the sound and video equipment used to conduct live and hybrid events such as lectures and presentations.
Network specialist	Keep computer networks running efficiently for their organization. They work within the IT department to test systems, perform maintenance, and troubleshoot local and wide area networks and Internet systems.
Learning management platform expert	Provides technical leadership in support of the institution's learning management system.
Instructional designer	Provides faculty with course design support in creating effective and engaging learning environments informed by desired learning outcomes. For example, providing guidance on designing accessible learning experiences.
Help desk staff	Provides technical support to users by researching and answering questions, troubleshooting problems, and guiding clients through corrective steps.

of technologies interacting with one another to create an effective learning environment (see Figure 17.1). These technologies are maintained and optimized by various technology professionals. "Technology professionals" is an umbrella term describing different technology-associated roles, such as AV professionals, network specialists, learning management platform experts, instructional designers, and help desk staff, to name a few (see Table 17.1 for job descriptions). While there are various technology professional roles, these are not uniquely ascribed to specific individuals. For example, the instructional designer might also be an LMS expert while providing AV support for faculty. While there is specialization, there is a lot of crossover in technology roles. This creates confusion around the roles of technology professionals and how they can contribute to medical education.[1]

The global lockdown that ensued because of the COVID-19 pandemic in 2020 brought technology professionals out of the shadows of medical education. Technology professionals, who had remained on the periphery of medical education, were now critical to its success. From 2020 to 2022, technology professionals actively worked with medical education faculty to create and disseminate online medical education. Post-pandemic, as medical education reverts to more traditional educational formats, technology professionals are moving back into the shadows. Unfortunately, this obscures the role that technology professionals play in medical education every day.

In this chapter, we examine the role of technology professionals who work behind the scenes in:

- graphics and media development
- faculty training and support for various technology platforms
- technology troubleshooting, and
- instructional design.

We include the experiences of technology professionals Erin Barry and Anita Samuel to provide a first-person perspective of the tasks technology professionals engage in within the context of both undergraduate medical education and graduate medical education (GME). In addition, the clinician perspective is brought in by Andrea Barker, Michael Battistone, and Jason Weiner.

Technology in Medical Education: An Academic Perspective

Traditional face-to-face education has, historically, been prioritized in medical education.[2] While medical professionals use cutting-edge technologies such as artificial intelligence and virtual reality in patient care, technology adoption has been slow in medical education.[3] However, there is a growing demand, even an expectation, from learners for technology-enhanced medical education.

Medical students in the twenty-first century, categorized as Millennials or Generation Z, engage with technology more than prior generations.[4,5] They use various digital resources to support their learning, including videos (e.g., YouTube, Pathoma), quizzing mobile applications (e.g., Anki), note-taking, e-books, and productivity enhancing tools (e.g., OneNote, Notability), and social media.[6] Medical students use mobile apps to access medical education resources to better inform patient care, revise for courses, and prepare for presentations.[7,8]

Medical education spans two learning environments – the academic and the clinical. In the academic formal learning environment, faculty teach in the classroom, anatomy lab, simulated patient suites, and the medical school classroom. In the clinical spaces, faculty teach in the workplace, hosting clerkship rotations and GME. Teaching within the formal environments is generally supported by the technology infrastructure and support staff of the medical school.

Medical education literature indicates that online learning is as effective as traditional face-to-face learning.[9] A combination of online and face-to-face learning through blended learning is widely encouraged in medical education.[9] Online instructional tools in medical education have included online videos, PowerPoint presentations, virtual simulations, webcasts, webinars, videoconferencing, and ePortfolios. Medical education faculty have limited training using these tools and find themselves working in unfamiliar terrain. They may find it challenging to incorporate educational technology into their teaching and assessment.[1] However, using technology in education has become important because "when used right, technology can free up time and facilitate opportunities for health professions students and faculty to master skills like patient-centered care and teamwork – competencies that are at the heart of good medicine."[10] (p. 9)

Teaching with technology requires faculty to have expertise in content, technology, and pedagogy.[11] Faculty need resources and training to become familiar with various technologies and gain competence in effectively using them.[12] In addition, they need technology support to create, distribute, and manage digital assets and to help them integrate technology into their teaching.[1] Technology professionals assist faculty in creating instructional products, differentiating instruction, providing resources, matching methods and media to content and learners, providing organized content, and using theory to inform practice and faculty development.[13,14] These professionals assume the roles of eLearning builders, technology experts, researchers, and quality analysts.[15]

Technology professionals do more than "show how it works." They coach faculty suggesting the best ways to use technology to enhance learning. For example, they offer guidance about the design of presentation slides, including choice of colours and use of text, incorporation of student interaction within the lecture, and ideas for active learning strategies. If lectures are recorded, post-production media experts may be involved in editing and producing a quality lecture video. Different technology professionals might be involved in various aspects of educational delivery, but they are all equally crucial for successfully incorporating technology into medical education. As Erin's experiences illustrate, technology professionals aren't simply offering brief "do this" kinds of tips; instead, they are deeply considering the content, audience, and speaker so that the educational value of the session is maximized:

I was tasked with redesigning lecture presentations. I started by assessing why we were giving a particular session and built out the main takeaway points learners needed to know. From there, the lecture could be simplified into a shorter overview. The redesign of the slides included decisions on the choice of colours, fonts, wording, and using pictures instead of words. Additionally, I had to find ways to incorporate more interaction in the lectures through technology available at our institution or the chat function of the videoconferencing software we were using. Collaborating with the faculty member included reviewing edited slides for content accuracy, discussing how to incorporate interaction, and working within their sphere of comfort.

– Erin Barry

Technology in Medical Education: Clinician's Perspective

In the past, going back to when we were in elementary school, the teacher would show a movie in the classroom. I'm old enough to remember that there was a film projector set up and plugged in, and usually, there was one older, responsible kid that got to be the projectionist. They were set up to do it, but there wasn't much to do. If something happened, it was pretty easy to figure out you stop it, unspool it, and get it all back together. And for many years, it has been a variation of that. As a chief resident, the lecturer would come with their carousel of slides, and the most you'd have to do is either unjam a slide or change a bulb, and that was it. Now it has evolved to the point where you cannot manage without knowledge, awareness, and comfort with the technology. It's not as intuitive as it used to be, and you can make things a lot worse by trying to solve the problems on your own.

– Michael J. Battistone, Director of the Advanced Fellowship
in Health Professions Education, Evaluation
and Research and associate professor

As Mike's story illustrates, technology has evolved rapidly, and medical educators increasingly find themselves working in unfamiliar environments with technologies that seem to change daily. If the affordances of these technologies guide medical education, then technology professionals support faculty in using these technologies to help deliver effective educational experiences.

Technology professionals work closely with medical educators to understand the teacher's educational vision and explore ways for realizing this vision. This is a process of co-creation, one in which the goals and needs of the faculty intersect with the capability of the technologies available at the institution. Mike's experiences illustrate how successfully incorporating technology into medical education requires collaboration between technology professionals and faculty:

We wanted to develop an animated orthopaedics software that includes theme music and a cartoon that gets drawn on the screen. We reached out to our graphic design team. They set up a meeting and we talked about what we wanted. The design team collaborated with us and brought in their areas of expertise. They spoke of the product from a technical and artistic perspective and worked closely with us to achieve our goals. It was a partnership.

– Michael J. Battistone

While technology professionals often work very closely with faculty, their work is typically invisible to students and leaders. When students see an end product of a creative animation or attend an interactive video lecture, they recognize the faculty member's work. All too often, the contributions of the technology professional are unrecognized.

The clinical environments, however, function independently. They often do not have a lot of technology support and clinician educators in these environments have to depend on personal support resources. Consequently, clinician educators are often frustrated by the lack of technology support. If they want to use educational technologies in their weekly lectures, they have to acquire the skills themselves. They function, as both Mike and Andrea explain, as "Lone Rangers," working in isolation without professional support:[1]

As a clinician educator, when I have to give a lecture, I end up going into the lecture rooms at least a half hour before the start of the session just so I can make sure that my flash drive will be accepted, that everything is there and set up so that I can switch between screens if I need to.

– Michael J. Battistone

We've wanted to take the content from our recurring face-to-face based course and place it on a platform where our residents and students can easily access it and come back to the content later if they need to. But there isn't anybody who could do that for us and so if we want to be able to expand access to our content, it's on us to figure that out – to figure out what platform is available for us to use, how to use the platform, and then how to maintain it.

– Andrea M. Barker, Co-director of the Advanced Fellowship
in Health Professions Education Evaluation and Research
and adjunct assistant professor

While the support provided by technology professionals might be unacknowledged, the absence of technology professionals to support teaching endeavours in the clinical environment is immediately felt by faculty. Faculty realize that spending time on fine-tuning their technology skills takes time away from their content, requires additional training, and competes with sparse time resources. This has driven some faculty to give up on attempting any technological innovations as they need more support to implement them. As Mike admits:

> It becomes so overwhelming that I just don't do it. I stay with technologies like email that I am familiar with.

– Michael J. Battistone

Technology in Medical Education: Technology Professionals' Perspectives

> I was helping a faculty member the other day with her Zoom session. She was conducting the Zoom session, and everything was running smoothly until all of a sudden, she realized she could not record her session. As the technology professional, I needed to step in, diagnose the issue, and record the session for her. My assistance went beyond troubleshooting. I had to be present throughout the session to complete the recording for her. That is a technology professional assisting a faculty member. When a faculty member mentions that they want help with a videoconferencing session, we sit with them through that session if for nothing else but moral support. We are there as technology professionals so if anything happens, we're there to jump in and help them.

– Anita Samuel

This narrative illustrates how technology professionals prioritize the learning experience of students and the teaching experience of the faculty, and the cost of that prioritization. Society's expectations of faculty and technology have evolved. Students expect faculty to have technological expertise, and faculty experience much pressure to meet these expectations. Technology professionals leverage their expertise with technology to help alleviate this stress for faculty. The work of relieving that stress was keenly evident to Erin during the pandemic:

> Much goes into delivering a quality lecture that is not always seen and appreciated from the technology professional's side. When COVID hit and everything moved online, we had a chance to create new material and experiences that were more engaging for the learners. Especially early on, when most classes were online and were back-to-back lectures, finding that balance between lectures, activities, and small group discussions to keep learners engaged was a challenge.
>
> When we moved learners into small group discussions, the planning of material to be used in that discussion was needed. We also had to logistically figure out the software we were using and think about grouping. Should we keep them in the same small groups from other classes, or should we mix them up? In many

cases, we decided to mix them up and we started receiving feedback that they loved meeting members of their class that they had never met before.

Throughout this process I had to take into account the technological competence of the faculty members. Did they have the required knowledge to use outside software? Do they have the ability to multitask? They would have to work with any additional technologies we wanted to use and also be able to set up the screen to share slides, while also monitoring the chat and reacting to what students were saying.

– Erin Barry

Technology professionals put on different hats in their interactions with faculty. They are simultaneously technology professionals, adult educators, and counsellors. Technology professionals have to work with faculty who come with a wide spectrum of technological competence. To be successful, they need to meet the faculty member where they are cognitively and work with them from there. As adult educators, they serve the specific needs of their audience and address their immediate needs.

Some faculty members approach technology with a lot of trepidation. In these instances, technology professionals are called on to provide psychological support and reassurance. This was a big part of their role during the COVID-19 transition to online education.

Concluding Thoughts

Being technology support staff is a backstage position. This is not the position where the person gets the credit. And yet, the service they provide is absolutely essential. You could have the best teachers in the world. But if they can't get their content out to their learners, their expertise becomes pointless.

– Andrea M. Barker

In the technology-driven educational environment of the twenty-first century, the backstage work of technology professionals makes faculty shine onstage. Unfortunately, in addition to being largely unrecognized, there is a stigma surrounding the persona of technology professionals. Media-propagated images of the nerdy, socially inept tech worker with an office in the basement or large rooms of call-centre staff have exacerbated negative connotations of what technology professionals actually do. Moreover, current institutional power structures result in technology professionals functioning primarily in a support function, compared to realizing their true potential and abilities. In addition to recognizing the crucial contributions of technology professionals to medical education, the expertise of technology professionals should be leveraged for the benefit of faculty, students, and medical education as a whole.

Additional Reading

Cenkner, M., Sonnenberg, L.K., von Hauff, P., and Wong, C. 2017. Integrating the educational technology expert in medical education: a role-based competency framework [version 1]. *MedEdPublish*, 6, 79. https://doi.org/10.15694/mep.2017.000079

Pei, L., and Wu, H. 2019. Does online learning work better than offline learning in undergraduate medical education? A systematic review and meta-analysis. *Medical Education Online*, 24(1), 1666538. https://doi.org/10.1080/10872981.2019.1666538

Anderson, M.C., Love, L.M., and Haggar, F.L. 2019. Looking beyond the physician educator: the evolving roles of instructional designers in medical education. *Medical Science Educator*, 29:507–13. https://doi.org/10.1007/s40670-019-00720-6

References

1. Cenkner, M., Sonnenberg, L.K., von Hauff, P., and Wong, C. 2017. Integrating the educational technology expert in medical education: a role-based competency framework [version 1]. *MedEdPublish*, 6, 79. https://doi.org/10.15694/mep.2017.000079

2. Lawrence, L. 2022. When medical education moves online [Internet]. *ASH Clinical News*. Available from: https://ashpublications.org/ashclinicalnews/news/1762

3. Burke, H. 2022. Top 10 new medical technologies 2022. *Proclinical*, April 14. Available from: https://www.proclinical.com/blogs/2022-4/top-10-new-medical-technologies-2022

4. Oblinger, D., and Oblinger, J. (eds.) 2005. *Educating the Net Generation*. Brockport Bookshelf .

5. Povah, C., and Vaukins, S. 2017. Generation Z is starting university – but is higher education ready? *The Guardian*, July 10. Available from: https://www.theguardian.com/higher-education-network/2017/jul/10/generation-z-starting-university-higher-education-ready

6. Zheng, B. 2022. Medical students' technology use for self-directed learning: contributing and constraining factors. *Medical Science Educator*, 32(1), 149–56. https://doi.org/10.1007/s40670-021-01497-3

7. Nuss, M.A., Hill, J.R., Cervero, R.M., Gaines, J.K., and Middendorf, B.F. 2014. Real-time use of the iPad by third-year medical students for clinical

decision support and learning: a mixed methods study. *Journal of Community Hospital Internal Medicine Perspectives*, 4(4), 25184. https://doi.org/10.3402/jchimp.v4.25184

8. Sayedalamin, Z., Alshuaibi, A., Almutairi, O., Baghaffar, M., Jameel, T., and Baig, M. 2016. Utilization of smart phones related medical applications among medical students at King Abdulaziz University, Jeddah: a cross-sectional study. *Journal of Infection and Public Health*, 9(6), 691–7. https://doi.org/10.1016/j.jiph.2016.08.006

9. Pei, L., and Wu, H. 2019. Does online learning work better than offline learning in undergraduate medical education? A systematic review and meta-analysis. *Medical Education Online*, 24(1), 1666538. https://doi.org/10.1080/10872981.2019.1666538

10. Thibault, G. 2015. *Technology in Health Professions Education 2015 Annual Report* [Internet]. Josiah Macy Jr. Foundation. Available from: https://macyfoundation.org/assets/reports/publications/jmf2015_annual_report_webpdf-1546879072.pdf.

11. Greenhalgh, T. 2001. Computer assisted learning in undergraduate medical education. *BMJ*, 322(7277), 40–4. https://doi.org/10.1136/bmj.322.7277.40

12. O'Doherty, D., Dromey, M., Lougheed, J., Hannigan, A., Last, J., and McGrath, D. 2018. Barriers and solutions to online learning in medical education – an integrative review. *BMC Medical Education*, 18, 130. https://doi.org/10.1186/s12909-018-1240-0

13. Anderson, M.C., Love, L.M., and Haggar, F.L. 2019. Looking beyond the physician educator: the evolving roles of instructional designers in medical education. *Medical Science Educator*, 29:507–13. https://doi.org/10.1007/s40670-019-00720-6

14. Sugar, W.A., and Luterbach, K.J. 2016. Using critical incidents of instructional design and multimedia production activities to investigate instructional designers' current practices and roles. *Educational Technology Research and Development*, 64, 285–312. https://doi.org/10.1007/s11423-015-9414-5

15. Love, L.M., Anderson, M.C., and Haggar, F.L. 2019. Strategically integrating instructional designers in medical education. *Academic Medicine*, 94(1):146. https://doi.org/10.1097/ACM.0000000000002475

18 Program Administration Coordinators in Postgraduate Medical Education

RENÉE E. STALMEIJER, MARLIES HANSSEN-BUDE, AND JAMIU O. BUSARI

... and if we had asked the residents "what does Mrs. Hanssen-Bude do?", what would they have said?

– Renée E. Stalmeijer

That I was the one in the helicopter, who had an overview of the whole situation, a "Jill of all trades" where you could go with issues ranging from broken beepers to scheduling of outpatient clinics or even to blow off some steam on a difficult day.

– Marlies Hanssen-Bude

As this description illustrates, the work of program administration coordinators (PACs) is far reaching and highly varied; however, understanding the complexity of this role and how it came into being requires a brief history of medical education's graduate-level processes. Postgraduate medical education (PGME) is the phase of medical education where medical trainees further specialize in a defined domain of medicine. To qualify for PGME, medical trainees must have completed 3–6 years of undergraduate medical education (UGME). The foundation of PGME as we know it is linked to the pioneering work of William Osler and Abraham Flexner in the early 1900s. The first residency program for specialty training of physicians was created by Sir William Osler, a physician and founding professor at Johns Hopkins Hospital, bringing medical students out of the lecture halls during their training to the bedside of their patients.[1] Abraham Flexner was an American educator, and he published his eponymous report in 1910. The Flexner Report launched the first reform of medical education in the United States[2] and has had far-reaching consequences for the training of medical doctors. Especially in the USA, Canada, and the UK, the key elements of Osler's and Flexner's proposals included the need for a strong foundation in biomedical sciences in the preclinical stages of the curriculum. They also promoted the acquisition of experience in patient care through formal clinical clerkships within hospital settings.

In recent years, these traditions have undergone several changes, including the introduction of competency-based medical education (CBME) and training in the medical curricula of several countries.[3,4] These changes have led to profound reforms in the curriculum and anticipated educational outcomes of residency training programs. Furthermore, several problems related to these reforms have surfaced.[4,5] For example, adopting CBME and the accompanying educational principles regarding curriculum, assessment, evaluation, and accreditation has increased the scope, depth, and workload for residency program directors (RPDs). RPDs, who are also physicians, are responsible for developing the structure of residency programs and assuring the quality of residency training.[6] To alleviate RPDs from these added responsibilities, the PAC role was introduced.

Program Administration Coordinators in Postgraduate Medical Education

Over the past few years, the development and implementation of the roles and responsibilities of PACs has witnessed different trajectories and iterations specific to different medical specialties, settings, and countries.[7] Consequently, the job descriptions of PACs are diverse and sometimes unclear,[6] ranging from clerical tasks (e.g., rotation schedules, planning of performance meetings, creating onboarding information packages) to managerial tasks (e.g., project management, duty hours oversight, preparing accreditation activities).[7] Furthermore, in addition to managerial roles, PACs also provide support for a variety of (personal) issues experienced by residents, ranging from issues with scheduling, study progress, physical illness, and adverse events.[8,9]

Compared to similar positions in the UK and the Netherlands, the roles and responsibilities of PACs in the USA and Canada are more distinctly defined[10] and professionalized and involve the need for certification and licensing.[11] The Alliance for Academic Internal Medicine is an example of such a process, in which the role of PACs in the USA and Canada have been identified and formalized into a self-governing entity called the "Administrators of Internal Medicine."[12] Unlike the USA and Canada, however, the PAC role in European countries is not well defined or carved out as a distinct professional entity. For example, in the Netherlands, there is no specific PAC role defined from a workforce development perspective. Instead, the role is filled by medical secretaries with demonstrable secretarial and managerial experience and an obvious affinity for medical education. Nevertheless, what all these versions of the PAC role have in common is the support they provide to RPDs and their strategic position as the "first point of contact" for residents during their training.[7]

In this chapter, we highlight the indispensable role of PACs in helping to build the learning infrastructure in PGME. We will focus on how PACs help in managing PGME programs and describe their instrumental role in helping to build the psychologically safe learning environments that foster positive learning experiences for residents.[13]

Indispensable Support in an Ever-Changing and Complex System: The Perspective of a Residency Program Director on the Program Administration Coordinator Role (Jamiu O. Busari)

The curriculum of residency training programs is required to align with guidelines and regulations set up by local institutions, specialist boards, and professional societies or institutes. The current forms of instruction in PGME operationalized in frameworks such as CanMEDS and the Accreditation Council for Graduate Medical Education (ACGME) Core Competencies, emphasize the importance of modern educational theories and instructional strategies. These modern principles of medical education have had significant influence on residency training in several countries, resulting in a wave of medical education curricular reform in Europe, North America, and Australia.[14-21] Consequently, the development and implementation of PGME has become more complex, requiring more contributions from different professionals at different stages and in different domains of the trajectory of the training program. As a result, RPDs need to continuously manage various aspects of the program related to curriculum design, content delivery, and operational processes in residency training programs.

With the added complexities of curricular reform introduced by the implementation of CBME, RPDs are increasingly tasked with overseeing the ongoing changes in the professional training and welfare of future medical specialists. Their job also involves working with a diverse team of professionals whose roles vary from medical to nonmedical and/or administrative responsibilities. PGME is, at all times, a complex interplay between enabling safe and effective healthcare of patients and enabling learning trajectories of trainees. In performing these tasks, therefore, many RPDs work closely with their PACs, whom to many, their invaluable contribution to the residency programs are invisible or unknown. As Jamiu explains:

Marlies Hanssen-Bude was of immeasurable support to me during my period as RPD in my department. Her vast amount of experience was crucial in helping me navigate the administrative complexities within our organization. She was what I considered to be my operational co-pilot, in addition to being my on-the-job mentor and collaborator.

To manage this interplay, RPDs need to effectively manage all actors contributing to the educational process, i.e., curriculum design, content delivery, and operational processes in residency training programs. This requires an intricate understanding of how each of these individuals contributes to the success of resident training programs and how they are positioned within the continuum of residency training programs. Although an RPD may be keenly aware of each of the contributors, they only become visible to trainees when their proximity to educational or active learning processes increases. For example, in a specialty department of a teaching hospital, contributors to education include patients, RPDs, clinical educators, and nurses; while "invisible educational contributors" include staff secretaries, hospital administrators, department managers, or PACs. This word can be hidden from learners' awareness unless, as Jamiu explains, someone (in this case the RPD) makes sure it is highlighted:

I made it a point of duty to explicitly inform each resident entering our program who Marlies was and what her role entailed in our department. Clearly positioning her role as PAC in the department's organizational and operational structure was important to me, to ensure that she received the acknowledgment needed to perform her duty fully. There was no iota of doubt to anyone that Marlies and I worked as an operational unit during my tenure as RPD, and the warm relationship we had then still flourishes till today.

Working on the Cusp of Patient Care and Residency Training: The Perspective of a Retired PAC for the Pediatrics Residency Program at Zuyderland Medical Centre,* Heerlen, the Netherlands (Marlies Hanssen-Bude)

As a PAC, I combined the role of outpatient clinic coordinator with that of administrative support of the RPD and the paediatrics department. I really enjoyed this combination of roles because it meant that I was close

---

* Zuyderland Medical Centre is a large regional hospital affiliated to Maastricht University and the Postgraduate Training Region South-East Netherlands (OORZON); it offers undergraduate and postgraduate clinical training for health profession trainees, including medical trainees.

to the source of what was going on in the clinic with regard to patient care and the residency training. It was a lot to have to combine both responsibilities, but during meetings I was able to help signal issues that arose at the cusp of the outpatient clinic and the residency program. These could be issues related to how to ensure sufficient supervision during residents' outpatient clinics or signalling struggling residents.

I was one of the first points of contact for the residents; I was the one to send out the invitation for (their) job interviews, and I coordinated the onboarding process. I ensured that they received (digital) information folders with all the necessary information about practicalities, such as lockers and identification cards, and information about protocols, departmental rules, and regulations. Together with the RPD, I created the schedules for the onboarding meetings with their clinical supervisors, as well as for their performance reviews.

Although residents mainly came to me for help with all sorts of practical issues related to patient care or training, they also saw and approached me as someone that could listen to them when they needed to vent. My door was always open for them, and I enjoyed hearing their stories, learning about what they did in their spare time, seeing pictures of their children, but also hearing about when they were struggling. I offered a safe space. I couldn't really offer any help, but often it was enough for them to vent, have a coffee, and then go back to work. These interactions also aided us (i.e., the residents and me) to create mutual respect and understanding.

My main tasks were to offer clerical support to the RPD. I assisted in creating scheduling for residents, clerks, and their supervisors. But I also coordinated the schedules in the outpatient clinic and performance appraisals of residents. I was part of the departmental meetings in which residents' performance was discussed, and besides making the minutes of these meetings, I was always invited to share my impression on each resident.

Because of my work in the outpatient clinic, my fellow outpatient secretaries and I saw how residents managed their clinic and interacted with patients and their parents. The RPD actively invited me to share my impressions of residents. In that way, I assisted him in his role by providing him with an extra set of eyes and ears. But at the same time, my interactions with the RPD resulted in giving new residents extra time for their patient consultations during their first month so they could get the hang of things. Furthermore, because we saw growing backlogs of administrative tasks of residents, we together initiated bi-weekly "admin afternoons" where residents would be freed of patient care to do administrative tasks.

My collaboration with the RPD was built on mutual respect and trust; I was taken seriously and actively invited to share my opinion. We clearly were partners in the work. You do, however, notice that not all physicians treated me and my colleagues as equals. During my long career, which has also spanned other medical and professional fields, I have noticed the importance of senior members of the profession treating me and the work that I do with respect. Not only does this contribute to the extent to which a safe learning and working environment is experienced by everyone there, but it is also a strong message to the next generation. Respect needs to be modelled by senior physicians because residents, especially the junior ones, assimilate to the dominant culture.

My role was not centre stage, and I have deliberately chosen a career which was supportive to others. I enjoyed organizing things in such a way that everyone could do what they did best, that everyone could shine in their own way, and that things just ran smoothly. That was what made me happy: facilitating job satisfaction, working hard together while still being able to laugh together. But mutual respect, understanding, and being taken seriously are essential.

Shaping the Experienced Learning Environment and Climate: The Role of Program Administration Coordinators from the Perspective of an Educational Scientist (Renée E. Stalmeijer)

PACs are part of the fabric that enables the day-to-day practice of PGME through the clerical and managerial support they provide to RPDs. Through their work behind the scenes, PACs play an instrumental role in shaping the experienced learning environment and climate.[22-24] They impact not only the formal aspects of education like supervision schedules, teaching moments, and performance meetings, but also the informal aspects like being a first point of contact when a resident experiences issues related to training, patient care, or personal life.[9] To further unpack the influence of the role of PACs on the experienced learning environment and climate, we will explore the PAC's role in residents' organizational socialization and hidden curriculum, residents' well-being, and assessment. Finally, we will reflect on the critical role of RPDs (and physicians in general) in capitalizing on the role of PACs in practice.

Through several formal and informal processes, PACs are important contributors to how residents socialize into (new) departments and into their role within the landscape of healthcare practice into which they are training to become a full-fledged and knowledgeable member.

PACs have a clear role in the organizational socialization[25] of residents through their involvement in the onboarding process of residents, be it as a resource person, organizer of formal introductory programs, or as the one who introduces the resident to "the lay of the land." Notably, the extent to which even RPDs are aware of the potential of PACs in this process may be limited or implicit at best. A recent Dutch study looking into strategies used by RPDs to support organizational socialization of residents addressed the existence of a "formal introduction program" for residents, but not the administrative and organizational support enabling this program.[26] Furthermore, only the role of the healthcare team in organizational socialization was considered, not that of other supportive and administrative staff.[26] In other words, much of the PAC's work can be invisible, even to the RPDs that they support.

PACs are ideally positioned to provide both formal and informal information on the "lay of the land" of the hospital and the residency program within it, acting as guides to the residents' workplace learning.[27] Moreover, in their supportive role of translating PGME rules and regulations to PGME practice in the workplace, PACs are instrumental within the transmission of the formal, informal, and hidden curriculum.[28]

Through the situated nature of their role, PACs are often a "first point of contact for residents,"[6] and some are confronted with decisions similar to those that a gatekeeper may need to make: what are the concerns of the resident and do I need to involve someone else in this process?[9] PACs' roles in residents' workplace learning were recently explored more deeply by Aono et al.[8] Using the lens of professional identity formation, Aono et al. were able to describe seven different roles that PACs had in residents' training, among which included creating a safe(r) learning environment, addressing mental health issues, and facilitating residents' self-assessment and confidence. Aono et al. suggested that the non-hierarchical relationship with residents and the continuity of the PAC role enabled PACs to be more sensitive to changes in residents' performance and well-being.

Through her work as an outpatient clinic coordinator, Mrs. Hanssen-Bude saw how residents interacted with patients and their parents (probably) more frequently than the residents' supervisors. Her role as PAC ensured that she was uniquely situated to offer a perspective on residents' competence development. From the perspective of programmatic assessment in which measuring competence development should be approached longitudinally and built on numerous, diverse data-points,[29] the PAC perspective could be highly relevant. However, given that the non-hierarchical nature of the PAC in relation to trainees is one of the strengths that the role of PAC has to offer to PGME, giving them a formal role in assessment may have adverse effects.

However, capitalizing on the full potential of PACs within the context of PGME requires that the RPDs and the entire clinical teaching team actively involve PACs as valuable sources and guides of learning. As Mrs. Hanssen-Bude points out, she was invited to share her impressions of residents, to co-create scheduling, and to voice her opinions during department meetings. But this engagement was highly dependent on the RPD and other medical staff and their openness to including her. This is certainly not common practice.[8] Moreover, Mrs. Hanssen-Bude specifically voiced how the way in which she was approached by attending physicians rubbed off on residents. Therefore, capitalizing on PACs in PGME should not only be facilitated by RPDs but by attending physicians in general, especially if health profession educators and RPDs aim to further empower PACs within PGME.

Concluding Thoughts

The design, implementation, and appraisal of the training programs in PGME is a complex and continuous process that involves contributions from different professionals at different stages of the educational process and in different domains of the trajectory of residency training. Often, the relevance and specific responsibilities of these professionals contributing to education in graduate training programs are unclear and unknown to trainees and or even other professionals contributing to the same program. Therefore, having a better understanding of the roles of different professionals and where they are positioned in the continuum of the training programs is helpful for a better appreciation of their tasks.

In this chapter, we highlighted the role of PACs in PGME and their invaluable support to residency programs and RPDs. In a time where the introduction of large, educational innovations in PGME, like CBME and programmatic assessment, is putting higher demands on residency programs, the indispensable role of support behind the scenes of PGME deserves to be spotlighted. The PAC role, for example, was introduced in PGME because of the need to support and alleviate the administrative and managerial burden of RPDs directing PGME programs. However, while the introduction of PACs has been extensive in some settings, others are still seeking ways to define and formalize this role in their settings. Nickel et al.,[6] for example, advocated for development of a standardized job description framework of PACs.

Despite the centrality of the PAC to effective PGME, their visibility to the average trainee or bystander is often limited. Visibility in medical education often seems related to the proximity to the educational or active learning process. The supportive and indirect nature of the PAC role in relation to training seems to have the effect that only those that directly work with the PAC are aware of the (extent of their) role, unfortunately leaving this role invisible to most.

Without the PACs, RPDs could not do their job effectively. PACs aid RPDs in navigating the administrative complexities within PGME and healthcare organizations. PACs are also a valuable source and guide for residents, but truly capitalizing on their potential requires support, visibility, and, as voiced by Mrs. Hanssen-Bude, respect.

Additional Reading

Aono, M., Obara, H., Kawakami, C., Imafuku, R., Saiki, T., Barone, M.A., and Suzuki, Y. 2022. Do programme coordinators contribute to the professional development of residents? An exploratory study. *BMC Medical Education*, 22(1), 381. https://doi.org/10.1186/s12909-022-03447-y

Hu, W.C., Flynn, E., Mann, R., and Woodward-Kron, R. 2017. From paperwork to parenting: experiences of professional staff in student support. *Medical Education*, 51(3), 290–301. https://doi.org/10.1111/medu.13143

Nickel, B.L., Roof, J., Dolejs, S., Choi, J.N., and Torbeck, L. 2018. Identifying managerial roles of general surgery coordinators: making the case for utilization of a standardized job description framework. *Journal of Surgical Education*, 75(6), e38–46. https://doi.org/10.1016/j.jsurg.2018.07.003

References

1. Epstein, R.M., and Hundert, E.M. 2002. Defining and assessing professional competence. *Journal of the American Medical Association*, 287(2), 226–35. https://doi.org/10.1001/jama.287.2.226

2. Flexner, A. 1910. *Medical Education in the United States and Canada: A Report to the Carnegie Foundation for the Advancement of Teaching*. Carnegie Foundation.

3. Cooke, M., Irby, D.M., and O'Brien, B.C. 2010. *Educating Physicians: A Call for Reform of Medical School and Residency*. Jossey-Bass; John Wiley & Sons Ltd.

4. GMC. 2015. *Promoting Excellence: Standards for Medical Education and Training*. General Medical Council.

5. Bleakley, A., Bligh, J., and Browne, J. 2011. *Medical Education for the Future: Identity, Power and Location*. Springer.

6. Nickel, B.L., Roof, J., Dolejs, S., Choi, J.N., and Torbeck, L. 2018. Identifying managerial roles of general surgery coordinators: making the case for utilization of a standardized job description framework. *Journal of Surgical Education*, 75(6), e38–46. https://doi.org/10.1016/j.jsurg.2018.07.003

7. Fountain, D., Quach, C., Norton, D., White, S., Ratliff, S., Molteg, K., Heyduk, D., Roof, J., and Badurina, L. 2017. The perfect storm is on the horizon! *Journal of Surgical Education*, 74(6), e120–3. https://doi.org/10.1016/j.jsurg.2017.07.020

8. Aono, M., Obara, H., Kawakami, C., Imafuku, R., Saiki, T., Barone, M.A., and Suzuki, Y. 2022. Do programme coordinators contribute to the professional development of residents? An exploratory study. *BMC Medical Education*, 22(1), 381. https://doi.org/10.1186/s12909-022-03447-y

9. Hu, W.C., Flynn, E., Mann, R., and Woodward-Kron, R. 2017. From paperwork to parenting: experiences of professional staff in student support. *Medical Education*, 51(3), 290–301. https://doi.org/10.1111/medu.13143

10. TAGME. 2023. Training Administrator of Graduate Medical Education – History. Available from: https://tagme.org/about-tagme/history/.

11. Guyatt, G., Cook, D., King, D., Nishikawa, J., and Brill-Edwards, P. 1999. Evaluating the performance of academic medical education administrators. *Evaluation & the Health Professions*, 22(4), 484–96. https://doi.org/10.1177/016327899022034428

12. Alliance for Academic Internal Medicine. 2023. Administrators of Internal Medicine (AIM). https://hl.im.org/about/about-aaim/aim. Accessed 21 December 2023.

13. Gilfedder, K.R., Giacomo, C., Randall, J., and Wilson, G.L. 2018. Medical education manager: a title worthy of the description. *Cureus*, 10(9), e3373. https://doi.org/10.7759/cureus.3373

14. Australian Medical Council. 2024. National Framework for Prevocational (PGY1 and PGY2) Medical Training (2024+). Available from: https://www.amc.org.au/accredited-organisations/prevocational-training/new-national-framework-for-prevocational-pgy1-and-pgy2-medical-training-2024/.

15. Frank, J.R. (ed.). 2015. *The CanMEDS 2015 Physician Competency Framework. Better Standards. Better Physicians. Better Care.* The Royal College of Physicians and Surgeons of Canada.

16. Manthous, C.A. 2014. On the outcome project. *The Yale Journal of Biology and Medicine*, 87(2), 213–20.

17. Scheele, F., Teunissen, P., Van Luijk, S., Heineman, E., Fluit, L., Mulder, H., Meininger, A., et al. 2008. Introducing competency-based postgraduate medical education in the Netherlands. *Medical Teacher*, 30(3), 248–53. https://doi.org/10.1080/01421590801993022

18. Simpson, J.G., Furnace, J., Crosby, J., Cumming, A.D., Evans, P.A., Friedman Ben David, M., Harden, R.M., et al. 2002. The Scottish doctor – learning

outcomes for the medical undergraduate in Scotland: a foundation for competent and reflective practitioners. *Medical Teacher*, 24(2), 136–43. https://doi.org/10.1080/01421590220120713

19. Swing, S.R. 2007. The ACGME outcome project: retrospective and prospective. *Medical Teacher*, 29(7), 648–54. https://doi.org/10.1080/01421590701392903

20. ten Cate, O. 2017. *Competency-based postgraduate medical education: past, present and future. GMS Journal for Medical Education*, 34(5), Doc69. https://doi.org/10.3205/zma001146

21. WFME. 2003. *Postgraduate Medical Education: WFME Global Standards for Quality Improvement*. World Federation of Medical Education. Available from: www.fmh.ch/files/c2/data/pdf/wfme.pdf

22. Lombarts, K.M., Heineman, M.J., Scherpbier, A.J., and Arah, O.A. 2014. Effect of the learning climate of residency programs on faculty's teaching performance as evaluated by residents. *PLoS One*, 9(1), e86512. https://doi.org/10.1371/journal.pone.0086512

23. Silkens, M.E., Smirnova, A., Stalmeijer, R.E., Arah, O.A., Scherpbier, A.J., Van Der Vleuten, C.P., and Lombarts, K.M.J.M.H. 2016. Revisiting the D-RECT tool: validation of an instrument measuring residents' learning climate perceptions. *Medical Teacher*, 38(5), 476–81. https://doi.org/10.3109/0142159X.2015.1060300

24. Roff, S., and McAleer, S. 2001. What is educational climate? *Medical Teacher*, 23(4), 333–4. https://doi.org/10.1080/01421590120063312

25. Bauer, T.N., and Erdogan, B. 2011. Organizational socialization: the effect of onboarding new employees. In *APA Handbook of Industrial and Organizational Psychology, Vol 3: Maintaining, Expanding, and Contracting the Organization*, edited by S. Zedeck, 51–64. American Psychological Association.

26. Galema, G., Duvivier, R., Pols, J., Jaarsma, D., and Wietasch, G. 2022. Learning the ropes: strategies program directors use to facilitate organizational socialization of newcomer residents, a qualitative study. *BMC Medical Education*, 22(1), 247. https://doi.org/10.1186/s12909-022-03315-9

27. Stalmeijer, R.E., and Varpio, L. 2021. The wolf you feed: challenging intra-professional workplace-based education norms. *Medical Education*, 55(8), 894–902. https://doi.org/10.1111/medu.14520

28. Hafferty, F.W., and Castellani, B. 2009. The hidden curriculum: a theory of medical education. In *Handbook of the Sociology of Medical Education*, edited by C. Brosnan and B.S. Turner, 15–35. Routledge.

29. Schuwirth, L.W., and Van der Vleuten, C.P. 2011. Programmatic assessment: from assessment of learning to assessment for learning. *Medical Teacher*, 33(6), 478–85. https://doi.org/10.3109/0142159X.2011.565828

19 The Humans of Accreditation

JASON R. FRANK, SANDY TSE, JAYMIE WALKER,
AND LISA THURGUR

There is a ritual nature to an accreditation survey in our system. You prepare for it many months in advance, like a papal visit. You perform an introspective catechism on your program. You practise the rites before the day. You prepare your community to ensure they understand standards and related sacraments. You buy catering. You receive esteemed visitors, the high priests of medical education, the wise ones from out of town. You pore over your program and its many meanings. You receive blessings and sometimes need to perform penance. Afterwards, you feel purified, rejuvenated, redeemed even. Other times, more atonement is needed.

    – Jason Frank, clinician educator and Professor of Emergency Medicine

The word "accreditation" has a variety of meanings in health professions education (HPE). In this chapter, we explore the lived experiences of those involved in looking at the quality of planned training programs. Accreditation may be considered by many to be an administrative process, a necessary bureaucratic exercise, a tick box to be completed at regular intervals. Instead, we argue that accreditation is an essential element of the societal enterprise that is HPE. And accreditation is fundamentally a social and societal phenomenon involving countless people around the world. We try to bring those invisible humans of HPE accreditation to life.

We have come together in this chapter with a variety of experiences in accreditation in HPE. Lisa Thurgur was until 2023 an award-winning program director at one of the top-rated residency programs in Canada. She has participated in accreditation as a teacher and program director many times. Sandy Tse has been a program director for residency education and is now the Assistant Dean for Postgraduate Medical Education at the University of Ottawa in charge of internal accreditation reviews of all Ottawa programs. Jaymie Walker is a senior resident in general surgery at the University of Calgary training program. She recently experienced an accreditation visit to her program. Jason Frank worked as the Director of Specialty Education at the Royal College of Physicians and Surgeons of Canada for 30 years. One of his roles was overseeing accreditation from a national and international regulatory body perspective. We have lived all sides of accreditation – standards, administration, surveying, and being surveyed as a program leader, teacher, and trainee.

The Phenomenon of Accreditation

Accreditation is a special kind of program evaluation that looks at HPE quality. For this chapter, we use the definition of the International Health Professions Accreditation Outcomes Consortium (IHPAOC):

Accreditation in the health professions is the process of formal evaluation of an educational program, institution, or system against defined standards by an external body for the purposes of quality assurance and continuous enhancement.[1]

Accreditation is an examination of HPE in the microcosm of the local training site. On paper, a program is a planned series of experiences and instruction that relates back to a set of formal standards that govern the training. Made real, the program is a large, dynamic, socially constructed community of practice. The practice, in this case, is learning to become a competent and compassionate health professional.

Accreditation systematically looks at the instructional activities, the teachers, and the learning environment of a local institution. Experts review the program to ensure that it is aligned with the defined standards. Ideally, these standards are created by the same professional community and all its participants. Standards are educational values articulated: written statements that express the instructional ideals of a community. Accreditation's magic lies in the thoughtful dialogue between expert reviewers and the leaders of a program around the application of the standards that leads to continuous improvement in program quality.

The literature of HPE accreditation is a small body of papers. To date, the majority of papers describe innovations in accreditation or associations between accreditation and various outcomes. The announcement of a new competency-focused system by the Accreditation Council of Graduate Medical Education (ACGME) in the *New England Journal of Medicine* in 2012 represents the former.[2] The works by Marta van Zanten and others document the impacts and importance of accreditation in

HPE.[3] What is missing from the published literature is the voices of those who conduct accreditation and those who are accredited. Accreditation bodies may hear a loud chorus of these stakeholders, but it is nearly absent from scholarly discourse. This chapter seeks to address this in some small measure.

The Experience of the Accreditor

> *A steward of an accreditation system feels the weight of the world on the shoulders. On the one hand, you serve all the learners in the system by ensuring that they get a quality experience, that they are kept safe in their learning environments, that they feel heard. On the other hand, you must craft standards and processes that are not so burdensome to the system that it causes harm. Ideally, any participant in an accreditation system sees it as fair and effective. You can sleep at night if the system makes training better, protects learners, rewards good teaching, and ultimately helps patients.*
>
> – Jason Frank

An accreditation system has a number of design elements. Accreditors facilitate continuous discussions among the community about these features so that the system is fit for purpose in HPE. Does the system emphasize quality assurance, continuous improvement, or both? Does it involve episodic reviews or ongoing oversight? How often are the accreditation standards reviewed? Do the standards focus on processes or outcomes? How are reviews communicated? What kind of authority does the accreditor possess to drive improvement? The design and operations of an accreditation system have the potential to impact everyone involved in HPE.

Since many accreditation systems have the ability to impose conditions on institutions and programs, accreditation can be consequential. Accreditation, when it works well, can stimulate changes to curriculum and learning environment. Accreditation, when significant problems are found, can change the careers of those involved. Accreditation protects trainees from bad training and the public from unprepared graduates. The accreditors therefore must be mindful of all of these impacts as they facilitate the workings of oversight of HPE.

While most of those involved in a training program will have experienced accreditation at some point in their careers, few can name the curators of the system. The accreditor has a position of authority, of leadership, of stewardship, and of significant responsibility. Who are these accreditors? They vary across jurisdictions and even within countries. In some countries, federal or state governments have an accreditation function. Other jurisdictions have ad hoc or formal non-governmental or academic regulatory bodies. Therefore, accreditors can be peer professionals with experience in HPE leadership and standards, or they may be a policy advisor to a government, or they may be a PhD-trained educational expert. Accreditors typically set standards at arm's length from the institutions seeking accreditation, gather data on these programs on site or on paper, and meet to assign an accreditation status.[4] The accreditor is a genus with many species.

The Experience of the Institutional Champion for Accreditation

It takes a village to have a good accreditation process. Programs understand that accreditation matters but everyone leaves it to the last minute. There is a significant amount of support needed to help programs prepare for a review. Everyone needs to understand what the standards mean and how they look in real life. The big message is that building a robust internal process requires engagement of programs, peer reviewers, and experts for continuous improvement.
    – Sandy Tse, Assistant Dean for Postgraduate Medical Education,

In the ecosystem of HPE accreditation, it is the local champions who are unsung heroes. These are institutional leaders who oversee an internal review process in advance of an external accreditation review. Thoroughly immersed in the standards of accreditation, these champions nudge all participants to prepare, conduct reviews, and coach communities to continuously improve instructional quality. Peer review is fundamental to their work: they organize members of the local community to visit their counterpart programs. Months ahead of external reviews, they ensure every aspect of the local institution is examined and thoughtfully communicated. To a great extent, the success of local programs and the accreditation enterprise overall depends on local champions to focus the attention of their local communities.

Internal accreditation leaders are heroic generals of HPE. They have the thankless job of pushing other (sometimes reluctant, always overburdened) educational leaders to conduct a self-study, looking at their own programs against the current standards for accreditation. They coach their colleagues to assemble evidence of their program's achievements and help them to rectify local educational gaps prior to an external review. They help prepare strategies. They practise the review process with their community of educators. They help to deploy armies of teachers. It is the internal accreditation champions that truly prepare institutions and programs for the process.

The Experience of the Program Director in Accreditation

Accreditation for a program director is the most rewarding, eye-opening, and self-reflective experience that you really only want to do every seven years. It is the epitome of the growth mindset, and despite the long journey of preparation and hard work that is involved, it is the best chance a program has to better themselves, for the good of the learners, the faculty, and the program as a whole.
> – Lisa Thurgur, previous residency program director
> and assistant professor

The program director is the most responsible academic officer for a given accredited program. They oversee all aspects of a local training community. They need to juggle the needs of learners, the program's teachers, and all the program's affiliated institutions. They need to recruit and select trainees, coach trainees in their development, police the professional behaviour of all involved in the training and design all aspects of the local curriculum. They need to be program evaluators, resident advocates, mentors, coaches, role models, clinicians, and great teachers. The program director is expected to be superhuman on a daily basis. And all of this work is expected to be done within their role; there is usually no extra compensation for the continuous quality improvement of a program.

In accreditation, the program director plays the leading role, and it is one of the key tasks of anyone in the position.[5-7] The program director prepares by reviewing the latest accreditation standards and engages the program community in a self-study. An accreditation submission is prepared, detailing the current state and future plans for the program in relation to the standards. This is all in addition to the program director's regular work and can be daunting. For a program director, accreditation can be intense, feel threatening, and be perceived as a high-stakes judgment on their abilities. Those who are strong in the program director role are gifted educators who recognize the accreditation process as an opportunity to reinvigorate their programs and connect with their local community.

The Experience of the Trainee in Accreditation

When you are a trainee, accreditation is a complex process that is difficult to comprehend. There are a lot of misunderstandings about what the process is for. There is a fear of failing, a fear of not being up to par. Trainees are already so busy and tired that taking the time to learn about accreditation is often not prioritized. There is a lot of pressure to perform well in residency in general, and accreditation is no exception. Accreditation is also an excellent time for trainees to reflect on all aspects of their program to identify gaps or issues we may have and discuss them with our leaders to try and provoke change. Overall, accreditation is an intimidating opportunity.

– Jaymie Walker, senior resident in general surgery

For trainees, accreditation can be baffling. The norms and procedures for accreditation are often experienced once during the training period of most learners. While immersed in their program, they may not be familiar with the accreditation expectations for all such programs. Trainees may not be clear what their role in accreditation truly is.

When accreditation works well, the learner's role is a critical one.[8] Trainees "live" the realities of the local curriculum and the learning environment. They can provide authentic insights into what is working and what is not. However, learners experience a power differential in educational ecosystems and may feel intimidated. In struggling programs, they may even be asked to withhold key information that would provide crucial evidence for the accreditation process, thereby undermining the value of accreditation and denying their voice. Learners without extensive experience with accreditation may not know what to say that can be helpful or generalizable, causing program leaders to fear the impact of comments they see as outliers. Accreditation works best when thoughtful learners work to enhance and improve their programs, empowered by the process of accreditation and anchored in the standards for their program.

Concluding Thoughts

Accreditation is considered an essential element of an HPE system, yet we have only limited research exploring the issue, and those involved are seldom given a thought by HPE communities. Accreditation impacts everyone. It engages and has implications for governments, regulators, education leaders, front-line teachers, and all our learners. Ultimately, as a process upholding quality and improvement, it impacts all the patients seen by all the HPE graduates in the world. For such a far-reaching enterprise, it has received proportionately little attention in our scholarly writings.

The people closely involved in HPE accreditation are diverse in their backgrounds and expertise – from education leaders, trainees, trainee union representatives, administrators, educationalists, policy analysts, and support technicians to decanal and institutional heads. Some are formally trained to contribute to the process, some are there as part of their formal titles, some are there for their lived experiences. All are essential ingredients in a large enterprise.

Like other forms of peer review, accreditation is fundamentally a human enterprise. It invokes emotions such as pride and despair. It generates work, reveals maltreatment, and celebrates educational achievement. Accreditation can be vilified and criticized for its flaws. It can also be honoured as a driving force for progress.

The humans of accreditation – all those who participate in the HPE training communities – are sometimes invisible. Accreditation, a formal enterprise of quality assurance and continuous quality improvement, can be experienced as intense, intimidating, or rejuvenating. Accreditation aspires to protect learners and improve learning. It is fundamentally a human endeavour designed ultimately to benefit HPE learners and their patients.

Additional Reading

Tackett, S., Zhang, C., Nassery, N., Caufield-Noll, C., and van Zanten M. 2019. Describing the evidence base for accreditation in undergraduate medical education internationally: a scoping review. *Academic Medicine*, 94(12), 1995–2008. https://doi.org/10.1097/ACM.0000000000002857

Frank, J.R., Taber, S., van Zanten, M., Scheele, F., and Blouin, D. 2020. The role of accreditation in 21st century health professions education: report of an International Consensus Group. *BMC Medical Education*, 20 (suppl 1), 305. https://doi.org/10.1186/s12909-020-02121-5

References

1. Frank, J.R., Taber, S., van Zanten, M., Scheele, F., and Blouin, D. 2020. The role of accreditation in 21st century health professions education: report of an International Consensus Group. *BMC Medical Education*, 20 (suppl 1), 305. https://doi.org/10.1186/s12909-020-02121-5

2. Nasca, T.J., Philibert, I., Brigham, T., and Flynn, T.C. 2012. The next GME accreditation system – rationale and benefits. *New England Journal of. Medicine*, 366, 1051–6. https://doi.org/10.1056/NEJMsr1200117

3. van Zanten, M., McKinley, D., Durante Montiel, I., and Pijano, C.V. 2012. Medical education accreditation in Mexico and the Philippines: impact on student outcomes. *Medical Education*, 46(6), 586–92. https://doi.org/10.1111/j.1365-2923.2011.04212.x

4. Taber, S., Akdemir, N., Gorman, L., van Zanten, M., Frank, J.R. 2020. A "fit for purpose" framework for medical education accreditation system

design. *BMC Medical Education*, 20 (suppl 1), 306. https://doi.org/10.1186/s12909-020-02122-4

5. Bing-You, R.G., Holmboe, E., Varaklis, K., and Linder, J. 2017. Is it time for entrustable professional activities for residency program directors? *Academic Medicine*, 92(6), 739–42. https://doi.org/10.1097/ACM.0000000000001503

6. Mainiero, M.B. 2003. Responsibilities of the program director. *Academic Radiology*, 10(1 suppl), S16–-20. https://doi.org/10.1016/S1076-6332(03)80144-7

7. Yager, J., Anzia, J.M., Bernstein, C.A., Cowley, D.S., Eisen, J.L., Forstein, M., Summers, R.F., and Zisook, S. 2022. What sustains residency program directors: social and interpersonal factors that foster recruitment and support retention. *Academic Medicine*, 97(12), 1742–5. https://doi.org/10.1097/ACM.0000000000004887

8. Professional Association of Residents of Ontario. nd. Accreditation. Available from: https://myparo.ca/accreditation/.

20 A Worker Betwixt and Between, Often Unseen: The Role of the Faculty Developer in Health Professions Education

RHODA MEYER, LIEZL SMIT,
AND SUSAN VAN SCHALKWYK

Faculty development is a slippery concept that is understood differently in different countries and contexts. Its programs have been described as "complex and heterogenous,"[1] (p. 832) with many aspects of faculty development – including how it is practiced, who is responsible for it, and where it is positioned in an institution – all playing out quite differently across the world. In addition, there exists a range of terms (such as "academic development," "staff development," "professional development," and "teacher training") that are used, often interchangeably, to refer to facilitating the professional learning of people in academia with an education-related responsibility.[2-4]

While the term "faculty development" appears to have support internationally in a health professions context,[1,3,5] definitional clarity is further challenged because of the way in which the field continues to evolve. The focus and intent of faculty development has shifted over time, much in keeping with perspectives on health professions education (HPE) itself, moving from a focus on skills development to an approach that considers the individual's professional identity formation and their professional learning.[2] The professionalization of the teaching role coupled with increasing demands being placed on academic faculty has catalyzed institutions to recognize their responsibility in providing the necessary support for these faculty – thus foregrounding the faculty development function and emphasizing its relevance in the context of health professions and medical education.

For the purposes of this chapter, we draw on Steinert's[6] (p. 4) definition that "faculty development refers to all activities health professionals pursue to improve their knowledge, skills, and behaviours as teachers and educators, leaders and managers, and researchers and scholars, in both individual and group settings." We recognize a broad audience is involved in and impacted by this work, including health professionals with an academic and/or teaching remit, faculty members, clinical educators, and so forth. We explore faculty development from the perspective of the faculty developer (Rhoda Meyer), the often-invisible worker who has the responsibility for creating the space within which professional learning pursuits may occur. In addition, we share insights from a medical specialist (Liezl Smit), someone whose journey as clinical educator has been influenced by the activities of such faculty developers, to emphasize why faculty development is important, why it needs to be affirmed and acknowledged, and why it needs to be seen. Rhoda starts our narrative with her story.

Who Is the Faculty Developer?

At my institution, I lead the faculty development portfolio in a centre for HPE. This is not a role that I was specifically trained for. I was trained as a healthcare professional, a nurse. I am also a health professions educator who has taught at higher education institutions for a number of years – including as a clinical teacher at various hospitals. My interest in matters education-related led to a master's in HPE followed by a PhD which focused on the learning environment. I have always enjoyed teaching and felt confident in the role. When I joined the centre and was given the faculty development portfolio in addition to postgraduate teaching responsibilities, I assumed that assisting others to "strengthen their teaching practice" would be relatively straightforward. This was, however, not the case. I soon realized the complexity of my new role. Even though I took over a relatively established faculty development program of orientations, workshops, journal clubs, and the like, I recognized that the prevailing literature was calling for faculty development to move beyond a "tips and tricks" approach to one that was more all-encompassing. It was not just about providing planned sessions to "teach" faculty how to teach, it called for more – for nurturing a culture where learning, teaching, and scholarship are affirmed, and creating an enabling environment (not unlike those I focused on in my doctoral studies) where faculty can flourish. Most importantly, this new mantle I had taken on meant that I would have to engage in a liminal space, betwixt and between, being both within the academic community on the one hand as postgraduate educator and supervisor while working in service of that community on the other. Although my role as lecturer felt legitimate and acknowledged by this community, the faculty development work was given less credence, sometimes felt unacknowledged – often invisible in the context of the teaching and clinical activities that characterize HPE. Achieving the credibility that can bring about more visibility of the faculty development role and the work that my colleagues and I do is an important and ongoing endeavour.

– Rhoda Meyer, Faculty Development Lead

Who is the "faculty developer"? Who typically takes up this role and where does the role fit within an institutional structure? How are faculty developers seen within our institutions? We do not easily find answers to these questions in the literature, which provides some justification for including a focus on this cadre in a book on the "invisible workers of medical education." However, Rhoda's story offers some insights that we can explore. As early as 2011, O'Sullivan and Irby[7] described a need for greater attention to who is doing faculty development work, while a 2016 systematic review of faculty development initiatives indicated that "no particular portrait of faculty developers" could be found, highlighting a lack of studies that have "examined the unique blend of skills and attributes"[8 (p. 780)] they require. In addition, faculty developers appear to be positioned in many different ways within institutions, with some having academic or faculty appointments and others falling into a professional or support staff environment including instructional designers, evaluation specialists, professional coaches, mentors, and the like. A growing trend is the establishment of centres or units of medical education or HPE that are situated within a school or faculty of medicine and/or health sciences. In many cases, these entities will be responsible for faculty development work but may also have a strong focus on scholarship, offering master's and PhD programs. Staff in these centres who are responsible for faculty development, such as described in the vignette above, may also fulfil a role as supervisor within these postgraduate programs, emphasizing their academic or scientist role.[9,10]

This brings us back to the individual faculty developers themselves. In health professions and medical education, those in a faculty development role typically come from a wide range of backgrounds. These can include "educationalists" with a strong educational research profile and no clinical background, on the one hand, and clinicians who have opted to engage in further education-related studies on the other. It is, however, not uncommon for clinicians or biomedical scientists to also contribute to this work. While some may have formal appointments, others can have a secondary, part-time, or even informal appointment as faculty developer,[11] building on the principles of peer and community learning. And there are many other variations in between. This inevitably has implications for the professional identity formation of a faculty developer, including the extent to which individuals own the relatively loosely understood role and their practice within it. It can also serve to make the role less visible.

Being in a "Liminal" Space

Susan is an example of someone who came to HPE with a higher education background. She has previously described the experience of becoming a faculty developer in the HPE context as akin to living a "chameleon-like existence" marked by border crossing as she sought to navigate between the different disciplinary discourses (such as the biomedical and the educational) and the professional cultures that she was trying to help others make sense of.[12] It is a complex, liminal space where faculty developers have been described as "betwixt and between,"[13] [(p. 203)] echoing Rhoda's earlier words. Faculty developers need to be flexible and able to adapt. They need to "read a room" and be sensitive to, and respectful of, the cultural and disciplinary norms and values represented within it. In addition, it could be argued that while the term "development" speaks to growth, it can also suggest that one is not good enough and therefore needs to be developed. This can place the faculty developer in an invidious position when established professionals (including faculty members, clinical educators) are invited, encouraged, and sometimes even required to attend or participate in an initiative aimed at their "development" and who might find themselves in positions of uncertainty, engaging with education-related ideas that feel alien and obscure.[14]

But of course, this all depends on who the faculty developer is, how they understand their own identity, and what their professional background might be. In addition, faculty developers tend to work at the nexus – what Whitchurch has called a "third space"[15] – between institutional imperatives (i.e., educational goals, curriculum initiatives, modes of teaching), institutional cultures that often determine the extent to which educational activities are valued and recognized, and the individual's own career goals. This can lead to tensions between faculty developers and the people with whom they work as they seek to mediate between the individual and the institution in a space characterized by issues of power and status, where there can be disciplinary contestation.[16]

Unique Blend of Skills and Attributes

What makes up the unique blend of skills and attitudes needed by a faculty developer? One of the challenges in trying to pin these down relates to faculty development's expanding remit, referred to earlier in the chapter. In many contexts, faculty development activities are characterized by workshops, sometimes as a series or a short course, as a key mode of engagement. These can be supported by, for example, consultations, journal clubs, lunchtime sessions, webinars, classroom visits by peers or educationalists, and mentoring.[2,8,17] Each of these activities need to be conceptualized, designed, developed, and ultimately implemented. This requires thoughtful planning and careful attention to detail on the part of the faculty developer and the faculty development team. This work often generates a significant administrative burden – work that the faculty developer may or may not have support for. This again signals a place of invisibility when managers and leaders do not understand the extent and nature of the work.

However, designing, planning, and implementing a range or program of activities is only part of the faculty development role. There are, for example, growing calls for greater accountability and for evaluating the efficacy of faculty development work.[18] In addition to this, faculty development is embracing an expanding remit of facilitating the professional learning of academics for their role not only as teachers, but also as educational leaders and scholars. In response, faculty developers are having to adapt and extend their own learning and scholarly growth. The "unique blend of skills and attitudes" has to be informed by educational theory on the one hand and craft knowledge on the other. As Rhoda explains, this is yet another layer of invisible work that needs to be completed by the faculty developer:

Skills related to leadership, research, and supervision have become important for the modern-day health professions educator. I would like to believe that my work as a faculty developer is informed by evidence. This includes insights from my scholarly work undertaken through research, the scholarly work of others in the field, and guidance from more experienced colleagues whose perspectives have also shaped the way I approach faculty development and the way I function within this role. The implication of all of this, however, is that as the faculty developer I first need to acquire these skills before I can facilitate the development of others. Time and opportunities for me to explore the field of faculty development through collaboration and research are critical to my own development as a faculty developer. Being and becoming a faculty developer is a lifelong learning experience.

– Rhoda Meyer

Faculty Developers as Agents of Change

Faculty development is ultimately about change – change in thinking that catalyzes a change in practice.[19,20] The role of the faculty developer, therefore, is being an agent of that change. For change to occur, work is needed to first facilitate awareness, then understanding, then acceptance, and eventually a different way of being and doing.[21] Work of this nature is, however, not easy, and it could be argued that it might indeed be invisible across an institution. It must take place amid a myriad of complexities: at the level of the individual faculty member who may or may not be engaging voluntarily and whose existing practice is being challenged; at departmental level where practices might be entrenched and there is little time to question them; and at institutional level with the issues of culture described earlier. Echoing Steinert, O'Sullivan, and Irby,[22] we argue that awareness across the personal, the relational, and the contextual is needed.

Writing from a higher education context, Peseta[23] (p. 65) has foregrounded an additional role for academic (faculty) developers that moves beyond that of being designer, planner, and implementer of activities to strengthen educational practices to one in which they embrace their stewardship in the field to have agency and "speak truth to power" – for example, to disrupt the traditional privileging of research above teaching that is complicit in making faculty development work less visible. Doing so, however, is incumbent on the faculty developer having credibility among those with whom they seek to work. Such credibility comes from being relevant and current in terms of what is happening in the field and engaging with scholarly work that can contribute to that field. Challenging entrenched institutional, professional, and disciplinary practices and cultures, however, needs to be done with extreme sensitivity on the part of the faculty developer, mindful of the borders they might be seeking to cross, mindful of those with whom they must work – many of whom themselves live betwixt and between their clinical commitments and their academic and teaching activities.

A Clinician's Perspective on Faculty Development

As a paediatrician working at a tertiary hospital, I have a dual appointment with both a government department of health and a school of health sciences. Each has its own priorities. For the department, it is service delivery and strengthening the health system. "Patients first" is its unwritten rule. For the school, it is student success and thus a focus on teaching, curriculum development, assessment, and research supervision for both undergraduate and postgraduate medical students. On a daily basis, I thus have to balance both my clinical practice and teaching while researching and publishing within my clinical discipline.

Patient care and health system strengthening is what I have been trained for. It has taken me six years of undergraduate studies and four years of specialist training, with an additional master's degree, diploma, and certificates along the way, to develop the expertise necessary to competently assess and manage my patients. Medicine, as an ever-evolving scientific field, necessitates me to continue to read, learn, and apply new knowledge and skills as I keep up with the latest developments. As such, I am required to provide annual proof of continuous professional development to maintain my licensure as a medical practitioner. In contrast, competency in teaching and learning was never part of my training and is not a requirement for practice – although I am aware that across the world, this is changing.

– Liezl Smit, medical specialist

In the context of HPE, faculty development is typically aimed at a diverse group of people – the broad audience referred to earlier – who may have competing interests and priorities. When the target is busy clinicians, these competing interests are compounded as people with established professional identities and often years of experience, coupled with demanding schedules, are encouraged to attend or participate in an initiative aimed at their development – an issue that, as we have seen earlier, can itself create tensions. The outcome of such exposure can manifest in many different ways, depending on: the extent to which the faculty member was concerned about teaching and therefore attended voluntarily, or not; the nature of the offering – whether it felt relevant; whether the teaching addressed a particular need; whether it was affirming of current practice; whether it offered the opportunity to engage with others; whether the attendee was supported by their environment, a head of department, or the like; and the context within which it occurred.[4,8] It also depends on the extent to which faculty development work is visible, a visibility that Liezl describes as having substantial impact on her very identity:

When I was appointed as lecturer at the university, I had to attend a university-wide faculty development workshop. I do not remember much of what was taught, or me translating what I had heard into practice. What I can remember is how disconnected I felt as I realized that teaching and research were the main responsibilities of most of my university colleagues outside the medical faculty. This was so completely different from my reality, where patient care was dominant and where teaching students in the clinical setting was far removed from the controlled classroom or laboratory setting. Fortunately, our Center for Health Professions Education offered several faculty development opportunities that spoke to my desire to become a better teacher and were cognizant of the context in which I teach. Through my interactions with our faculty development team, I realized that teaching and learning goes beyond a set of tips and tricks. They introduced me to the field of medical education and the body of scholarship underpinning the "what" and "how" of teaching, learning, and assessment. They created a space where I met like-minded clinicians with an interest in teaching and learning, and where we could share successes and challenges and learn from each other. These experiences made me reflect on and adapt my own teaching, learning, and assessment practices in the clinical setting based on evidence. I subsequently became involved in curriculum development and leadership/management opportunities. Faculty development related to teaching, learning, and assessment practices became part of my ongoing individual professional journey as clinician, educator, leader, and scholar.

– Liezl Smit

Why Is Faculty Development So Important?

Although hospitals and clinics are primarily designed for patient care and not teaching in the "traditional sense," this space is where medicine is practiced, and where students have the opportunity to apply and integrate their knowledge, skills, and values. Clinical training is thus a vital part of the medical curriculum, although undergraduate medical students often struggle to learn in this complex environment. My faculty development colleagues made me realize that both present student success and future patient safety are influenced by my ability to facilitate student learning in this setting. This makes my being prepared and equipped for my teaching role as important as staying abreast of my scientific field.

Most of my clinician colleagues unfortunately still do not seem to value the scholarship of teaching and learning and believe that no specific training or knowledge is needed to be an effective teacher. The faculty development opportunities on offer are also mostly taken up by those already interested in teaching, learning, and assessment. I see the same faculty members at these events, the curriculum committee meetings, and HPE conferences. Hopefully this will change in future as the need for faculty development becomes more visible, but for now those sharing my passion for teaching have become my community of practice as I journey towards becoming a better educator.

– Liezl Smit

In a 2011 editorial, Searle and colleagues[20] (p. 405) suggested that "if you want to change medicine, you have to change those who teach medicine" and that this required "quality faculty development." Some years later in another editorial, Sklar[24] (p. 1586) pointed to a "different frame" for faculty development that acknowledges the multiple identities of those who are involved in education-related activities in our institutions; that understands the need for lifelong learning and environments that create opportunities for growth; and that embraces the need for empowerment as part of its remit. This, he argued, could "lead to a healthier, more capable workforce of medical educators, researchers, clinicians, scholars, and administrators who would be able to anticipate and address the educational needs of their students and the healthcare needs of the public and, in so doing, also meet their full potential as individuals and faculty." This revision could have long-lasting and positive impact for educators who, as Liezl narrates, have had to find agency in the space between education and patient care:

> *I still introduce myself as a pediatrician with an interest in medical education. I have become adept at using the discourse of medical education when among those who value and nurture teaching and learning but switching to the language of natural sciences when among my clinical colleagues. The positive aspect of this dual position is the potential to strengthen the understanding and connection between education and medicine over time, in context, and through working with people, which is what faculty development is all about.*
>
> – Liezl Smit

Concluding Thoughts

As HPE continues to evolve, demanding ever more from those who have some form of educational remit, so too will the role of the faculty developer continue to expand – possibly becoming less "invisible" than might have been the case in the past. This will require foregrounding their work and enhancing credibility within their institutions. Leibowitz and colleagues[25] have argued that the perceptions that faculty hold of those responsible for enabling their professional learning, and the regard attached to the environment in which the faculty development responsibility is located, fundamentally influence its success. These perceptions are often coloured by institutional messaging with regard to recognition and reward for teaching, and the privileging of disciplinary research above teaching.[26] While the clinician-teacher identity is one that has been extensively documented,[22] the identity duality experienced by the faculty developer is still relatively unexplored, indeed invisible, in the literature. It is, however, quite possible that embracing this invisibility can serve as an enabler for bridging between domains. Whether it is the educational expert who must engage within a particular field or profession, or the healthcare professional who has taken on the mantle of faculty developer, or a variation thereof, all must navigate the liminal and often-invisible space betwixt and between institutional cultures, disciplinary imperatives, professional standing, and the individual's context and inner motivations.

Additional Reading

Sklar, D.P. 2016. Moving from faculty development to faculty identity, growth, and empowerment. *Academic Medicine*, 91(12), 1585–7. https://doi.org/10.1097/acm.0000000000001447

Steinert, Y. 2020. Faculty development: from rubies to oak. *Medical Teacher*, 42(4), 429–35. https://doi.org/10.1087300/0142159X.2019.1688769

Steinert, Y., O'Sullivan, P.S., and Irby, D.M. 2019. Strengthening teachers' professional identities through faculty development. *Academic Medicine*, 94(7), 963–8. https://doi.org/10.1097/ACM.0000000000002695

References

1. Proctor, D., Leeder, D., and Mattick, K. 2020. The case for faculty development: a realist evaluation. *Medical Education*, 54(9), 832–42. https://doi.org/10.1111/medu.14204

2. Leslie, K., Baker, L., Egan-Lee, E., Esdaile, M., and Reeves, S. 2013. Advancing faculty development in medical education: a systematic review. *Academic Medicine*, 88(7), 1038–45. https://doi.org/10.1097/ACM.0b013e318294fd29

3. Stes, A., Min-Leliveld, M., Gijbels, D., and Van Petegem, P. 2010. The impact of instructional development in higher education: the state-of-the-art of the research. *Educational Research Review*, 5(1), 25–49. https://doi.org/10.1016/j.edurev.2009.07.001

4. van Schalkwyk, S., Leibowitz, B., Herman, N., and Farmer, J. 2015. Reflections on professional learning: choices, context and culture. *Studies in Educational Evaluation*, 46, 4–10. https://doi.org/10.1016/J.STUEDUC.2015.03.002

5. Hafler, J.P., Ownby, A.R., Thompson, B.M., Fasser, C.E., Grigsby, K., Haidet, P., Kahn, M.J., and Hafferty, F.W. 2011. Decoding the learning environment of medical education: a hidden curriculum perspective for faculty development. *Academic Medicine*, 86(4), 440–4. https://doi.org/10.1097/ACM.0b013e31820df8e2

6. Steinert, Y. (ed.). 2014. *Faculty Development in the Health Professions: A Focus on Research and Practice*. Springer Science & Business Media.

7. O'Sullivan, P.S., and Irby, D.M. 2011. Reframing research on medical education. *Academic Medicine*, 86(4), 421–8. https://doi.org/10.1097/ACM.0b013e31820dc058

8. Steinert, Y., Mann, K., Anderson, B., Barnett, B.M., Centeno, A., Naismith, L., Prideaux, D., et al. 2016. A systematic review of faculty development

initiatives designed to enhance teaching effectiveness: a 10-year update: BEME Guide No. 40. *Medical Teacher*, 38(8), 769–86. https://doi.org/10.1080/0142159X.2016.1181851

9. Humphrey-Murto, S., O'Brien, B., Irby, D.M., van der Vleuten, C., ten Cate, O., Durning, S., Gruppen, L., et al. 2020. 14 years later: a follow-up case-study analysis of 8 health professions education scholarship units. *Academic Medicine*, 95(4), 629–36. https://doi.org/10.1097/ACM.0000000000003095

10. van Schalkwyk, S., O'Brien, B.C., van der Vleuten, C., Wilkinson, T.J., Meyer, I., Schmutz, A.M., and Varpio, L. 2020. Exploring perspectives on health professions education scholarship units from sub-Saharan Africa. *Perspectives on Medical Education*, 9, 359–66. https://doi.org/10.1007/s40037-020-00619-8

11. O'Sullivan, P.S., and Irby, D.M. 2014. Identity formation of occasional faculty developers in medical education: a qualitative study. *Academic Medicine*, 89(11), 1467–73. https://doi.org/10.1097/ACM.0000000000000374

12. van Schalkwyk, S., and McMillan, W.J. 2016. "I have a chameleon-like existence": a duo-ethnographic account of border crossing by two academic development practitioners. *South African Journal of Higher Education*, 30(6), 207–23. https://doi.org/10.20853/30-6-735

13. Little, D., and Green, D.A. 2012. Betwixt and between: academic developers in the margins. *International Journal for Academic Development*, 17(3), 203–15. https://doi.org/10.1080/1360144X.2012.700895

14. Adendorff, H.J. 2011. Strangers in a strange land – on becoming scholars of teaching. *London Review of Education*, November 1. https://doi.org/10.1080/14748460.2011.616323

15. Whitchurch, C. 2015. The rise of third space professionals: paradoxes and dilemmas. In *Recruiting and Managing the Academic Profession*, edited by U. Teichler and W.C. Cummings, 79–99. Springer

16. Green, D.A., and Little, D. 2013. Academic development on the margins. *Studies in Higher Education*, 38(4), 523–37. https://doi.org/10.1080/03075079.2011.583640

17. Clark, J.M., Houston, T.K., Kolodner, K., Branch, W.T., Levine, R.B., and Kern, D.E. 2004. Teaching the teachers: national survey of faculty development in departments of medicine of US teaching hospitals. *Journal of General Internal Medicine*, 19, 205–14. https://doi.org/10.1111/j.1525-1497.2004.30334.x

18. Boughey, C. 2022. Not there yet: knowledge building in educational development ten years on. *Teaching in Higher Education*, 27(8), 992–1004. https://doi.org/10.1080/13562517.2022.2121158

19. Bligh, J. 2005. Faculty development. *Medical Education*, 39(2), 120–1. https://doi.org/10.1111/j.1365-2929.2004.02098.x

20. Searle, N.S., Thibault, G.E., and Greenberg, S.B. 2011. Faculty development for medical educators: current barriers and future directions. *Academic Medicine*, 86(4), 405–6. https://doi.org/10.1097/ACM.0b013e31820dc1b3

21. van Schalkwyk, S. 2010. Early assessment: using a university-wide student support initiative to effect real change. *Teaching in Higher Education*, 15(3), 299–310. https://doi.org/10.1080/13562511003740874

22. Steinert, Y., O'Sullivan, P.S., and Irby, D.M. 2019. Strengthening teachers' professional identities through faculty development. *Academic Medicine*, 94(7), 963–8. https://doi.org/10.1097/ACM.0000000000002695

23. Peseta, T.L. 2014. Agency and stewardship in academic development: the problem of speaking truth to power. *International Journal for Academic Development*, 19(1), 65–9. https://doi.org/10.1080/1360144X.2013.868809

24. Sklar, D.P. 2016. Moving from faculty development to faculty identity, growth, and empowerment. *Academic Medicine*, 91(12), 1585–7. https://doi.org/10.1097/ACM.0000000000001447

25. Leibowitz, B., Bozalek, V., van Schalkwyk, S., and Winberg C. 2015. Institutional context matters: the professional development of academics as teachers in South African higher education. *Higher Education*, 69, 315–30. https://doi.org/10.1007/s10734-014-9777-2

26. Cleland, J.A., Jamieson, S., Kusurkar, R.A., Ramani, S., Wilkinson, T.J., and van Schalkwyk, S. 2021. Redefining scholarship for health professions education: AMEE Guide No. 142. *Medical Teacher*, 43(7), 824–38. https://doi.org/10.1080/0142159X.2021.1900555

21 Traversing the Desert in Search of Water: The Work of Wellness Champions in Medical Education

WILLIAM E. BYNUM, ANDRADA D. NEACSIU, AND JOSEPH A. JACKSON

Constance is a third-year medical student completing her clinical rotations. As she sits through a resilience development session, she bemoans yet another attempt by the school to seemingly fix what she increasingly feels is an environmental hazard: the impossibility of learning medicine, maintaining her wellness, and being herself. The rigours of medical school have forced her to cut back on her hobbies and invest less time in her relationships, and yet, she's still struggling to perform at the high level she expects of herself. This has left her questioning whether she's good enough to make it in medicine and feeling burned out.

Across the hospital, John, a first-year family medicine resident, is on the first day of his labour and delivery rotation. Lacking an understanding of the norms or culture of the unit, John feels uneasy expressing himself, particularly in what feels like an intimidating, hierarchical environment. After eight rotations (each with its own new set of learning curves), he's physically, mentally, and emotionally exhausted, and self-doubts about his competence and ability to fit in – especially as one of the only African American male physicians – abound. John has real concerns about how he is going to make it through this rotation and the remainder of intern year, and he is unsure about what to do with these feelings.

– William Bynum, Family Medicine Residency Program
Director and shame researcher

As these examples illustrate, learning medicine is an emotionally complex endeavour. Medical learners seeking self-actualization as independent physicians must navigate steep learning curves; must confront deficiencies in knowledge and skill; must engage in risk-laden learning behaviours; must endure identity threats and assimilation pressures; and must, nevertheless, fully engage with these realities while traversing the challenging learning environments in which they occur. The incredible growth and development that occurs during this long journey is long known. While confronting death, illness, inequity, and uncertainty, medical learners are trained to meet – and often exceed – their obligations to society through high levels of skill, competence, and altruism.

There is increasing awareness, however, of the many ways in which medical learners' well-being suffers during this long journey. Indeed, the many risks and challenges inherent in learning medicine, while growth-inducing, may promote psychological distress, mental illness, and identity dissonance in medical learners, ultimately undermining the goal of creating the skilled, competent, and altruistic physicians that our society needs.

Supporting the development and well-being of such future physicians requires, quite literally, the work – often invisible – of thousands: the individuals in medical education who support the well-being of medical learners and optimize the environments in which they learn. We are a team of three academic healthcare professionals whose roles – a residency program director (William Bynum), residency behaviouralist (Andrada Neacsiu), and medical student affairs dean (Joseph Jackson) – are visible, but whose work in support of learner well-being – which often occurs behind closed doors, after hours, and in the quiet recesses among the commotion of medical learning – is quite the opposite.

In this chapter, we outline what is known and unknown about the state of learner wellness in medical education and the environmental factors influencing it. We direct attention to a central argument: that supporting the well-being of medical learners requires *both* holistic support of individuals and environmental modification and reform. We then highlight the work of two individuals doing the invisible work of advancing learner wellness in medical education – a student affairs dean and a PhD-trained clinical psychologist serving as a behaviouralist in a family medicine residency program.

The Challenges of Supporting Learner Well-Being: An Academic Perspective

Over the past decade, a chorus of stakeholders – ranging from researchers to funding agencies to national action collaboratives – have directed significant attention to the crisis of impaired well-being in medical learners. Simultaneously, greater attention has been directed to the unique nature of the environments where learning occurs and the ways in which these environments may influence the well-being of the learners therein. In this section, we call attention to the intrapersonal, interpersonal, and environmental challenges that must be addressed in doing the work of supporting medical learner well-being.

Medicine attracts the world's brightest students. The educational pathways they must traverse to enter medical training are intense and require high levels of work ethic, sacrifice, and achievement. Many students enter medical training as highly accomplished students who have seldom failed or struggled academically. Other students have navigated pre-medical pathways filled with adversity, ranging from childhood trauma to socioeconomic instability to systemic racism. Still others arrive at the gates of medicine with pre-existing physical and/or mental illness. Accordingly, in passing through medicine's gates and into its educational institutions, students bring with them certain tendencies, characteristics, health conditions, and contingencies of self-worth, all of which are active – albeit potentially unrecognized – during medical learning.[1] Such tendencies may include possessing a fixed mindset, the tendency to compare to others, perfectionism, and performance-based self-esteem.[1,2]

Upon passing through these gates, medical students encounter academically, physically, and emotionally demanding learning environments for which they may be unprepared. For example, in a study on shame in medical students, many instances of shame and emotional distress were triggered by events related to normal learning processes, including struggling on a new task, being wrong in public, or failing to achieve a top score.[3] Intense workloads, the public nature of medical learning, and competition for limited resources (e.g., competing for residency slots) can incur significant performance pressure, require tremendous self-sacrifice, and prompt identity negotiation in students navigating medical school curricula.[3,4] Transition periods such as the start of a new clinical rotation or the beginning of internship may be particularly high-risk periods for intrapersonal distress as learners leave relationships behind, adjust to new institutional cultures, assimilate to environmental norms, and navigate steep learning curves.[5-7]

These challenges can be potentiated within suboptimal medical learning environments characterized by a lack of psychological safety, the presence of learner mistreatment, and/or pervasive disrespect.[8-10] A 2006 study highlighting the prevalence of problematic learning environments reports that 40 per cent and 84 per cent of graduating medical students reported being harassed and belittled, respectively.[11] Other studies reveal mistreatment in the form of verbal abuse, discrimination, sexual harassment, and even direct physical abuse.[12,13] The effects of mistreatment may be significant, including development of post-traumatic stress symptoms, depression, and suicidality as well as reduced confidence in clinical skills.[11,14,15] In qualitative studies, mistreatment is a pervasive trigger of damaging shame reactions in medical learners, leading to psychological distress, an impaired sense of belonging, and altered identity formation.[3,7] This presents a sobering and mystifying reality: learners must endure the risks of mistreatment and abuse while simultaneously navigating rigorous training demands and striving to become competent, empathic physicians.

It is against this backdrop that medical trainees manifest myriad forms of intrapersonal distress during medical training, including high rates of depression,[16] burnout,[17] stress,[18] and anxiety.[19] In what can be considered a public health crisis, these jarring levels of impaired well-being have spawned widespread attempts to support the mental health and well-being of medical learners, including duty hour limitations, stress management training, support group meetings, mindfulness interventions, curricular reform, and yoga classes.[20-24] Unfortunately, when evaluated, many such interventions have not shown statistically significant improvements in the dimensions of learner well-being (e.g., burnout) that they intend to improve.[21,25,26] For example, in a systematic review of interventions to address learner burnout, only 5 of 14 included studies showed statistically significant improvement in burnout scores, with one study showing a statistically significant worsening of burnout.[25]

The inconsistent effectiveness of these interventions raises two primary concerns that must be considered by stakeholders working to advance medical learner wellness. First, it is likely that the medical education community lacks a thorough and nuanced understanding of what it means to be well, or unwell, while learning medicine.[27] Further, the predominant focus on dimensions of impaired well-being that can be easily measured (e.g., burnout and depression) has contributed to narrow conceptualizations of what is an otherwise highly complex, multidimensional phenomenon.[27] Aspects of human experience that are more stigmatized, difficult to identify, and infrequently discussed (e.g., shame, trauma) may remain hidden and unaddressed within those narrow conceptualizations. Second, many forms of learner distress that leaders hope to solve may be normal and inevitable experiences within the context of today's medical learning environments.[27] For example, are we surprised that a resident working 80 hours per week, encountering daily human suffering, struggling to engage in self-care, and enduring suboptimal learning environments is burned out and/or depressed? Is it reasonable to expect and hope that they will maintain their wellness in the face of such realities? Focusing on solving learner impairment without addressing its underlying systemic causes (which may or may not be avoidable) may further entrench impaired well-being and miss opportunities for resilience development.[27]

Supporting Learner Well-Being: A Clinical Perspective and Moral Imperative

The work of supporting learner well-being has critical clinical implications for both learners and the patients they serve. The clinical effects of impaired well-being on learners can be severe, with suicide representing its starkest, most earth-shattering form. Likely resulting from an amalgamation of intersecting forces,[28] the occurrence of learner suicide is inconceivable, and yet it is a reality with which too many in medical education must grapple. Subordinate – and potentially antecedent – to suicide are numerous other effects of impaired well-being in medical learners, ranging from social isolation and impaired belonging to dysfunctional social relationships to substance abuse.[4,7,29,30] Such effects may pervade not only attempts to learn (e.g., through disengagement, avoidance, and cognitive dysfunction) but also efforts to maintain wellness, relationships, and personal identity outside of the medical learning environment. This combination may render medical learners particularly susceptible to the effects of their distress when they perceive failure in multiple areas of their lives.[7]

Impaired learner well-being can have significant effects on patients cared for in clinical learning environments. For one, nonadherence to basic physiological needs (e.g., sleep deprivation, lack of sufficient nutrition) may impair learner performance, judgment, and clinical decision making. In one study, neurocognitive performance on a battery of tests after a long call rotation was similar to finishing a short call plus consuming alcohol to a blood level of 0.05 per cent.[31] Emotional distress may indirectly lead to risk of harm as well. For example, the effects of shame, which often prompt attempts to hide and disengage,[4,7] may lead to errors of omission, failure to speak up in support of patient safety, or lacklustre diagnostic inquiry, each of which may carry downstream risk to patients.

Thus, given the situated vulnerability of learners – and the vulnerability of the patients who may be impacted by their distress – the provision of authentic, proactive, and dedicated support for their well-being is a moral imperative, one that must be executed while considering the inherent challenges to well-being that lurk in the environments in which they work and learn. In the following section, we highlight how two individuals – an associate dean of student affairs in a medical school and a clinical psychologist embedded in a family medicine residency program – meet this moral imperative, support the wellness of medical learners, and work towards meaningful environmental reform. Importantly, while both individuals clearly hold positions in support of medical trainees, it is the depth and breadth of their *work* in providing that support that is invisible.

Supporting Learner Well-Being: An Associate Dean of Medical Student Affairs Perspective

It is five days before Match Day when our Office of Student Affairs learns which students did not successfully match in their chosen specialty. One of the students I have advised for nearly four years is on this devastating list. After giving him a few moments to sit with the news, I reach out by phone to inquire about his safety and to invite him to my office to begin the process of identifying alternate plans.*

He shares his fears, disillusionment, and disappointment about having given so much energy and effort to a career from which he now hears, "You are no longer welcome here." Our early discussions prioritize attention to self-care and the practical steps that must be taken to move forward in the face of this painful rejection. In subsequent meetings over the weeks and months that follow, we continue to unpack this event, manage the emotional fallout, seek recovery, and reimagine his future.

– Joseph Jackson, Associate Dean for Student Affairs

As a student affairs dean in a medical school, I (Joseph) dwell in the crossroads of the beautiful yet distressing realities that meet my students as they navigate their medical school careers. My professional work focuses on enhancing and supporting student success – which is inextricably bound to student well-being – in the myriad ways it can be defined. While much of my work is public, the heart of it dwells in the realm of discretion and invisibility.

Most days start with scheduled one-to-one student advising meetings that always begin with a physical and mental health check-in. Some days begin with – and many nights are interrupted by – meetings to address a crisis: housing insecurity, financial distress, a family death, or a legal complication. In these meetings, students disclose their true selves and articulate the ways they have neglected their health, experienced the consequences of unhealthy lifestyles, or suffered from circumstances beyond their control. While some students master the art of balance and wellness integration, others plod or lurch forward, focused simply on surviving.

---

* Match Day in the United States is the day when graduating medical students learn where they have been accepted for residency training.

I am often the first person to hear about students in distress: the first to hear from faculty who are concerned about their students' well-being; the first to hear when law enforcement has interfaced with our students; the first to hear from a student who has received tragic news from family; and the first to hear about a student being mistreated in the learning environment. In the difficult – and often private – conversations that follow, I try to calmy reassure students and support an intact sense of self as they navigate real-life challenges that threaten its disintegration. I also interface with students as they struggle to meet their basic human needs. The high degree of focus placed on medical students' competence development often shields awareness of these struggles, such as difficulty accessing food, shelter, and clothing. Colleagues and administrators join me in the invisible work of supporting such students' needs. This work can encompass a myriad of activities, such as providing emergency loans, assisting with access to a stocked food pantry, and finding other faculty and staff who compassionately offer up their homes or financial gifts.

My workday also includes time supporting students through academic challenges that may have profound effects on their physical and mental health. In addressing academic struggle, I collaborate with students to navigate the anxiety of performing while learning, the shame of perceived failure, and the reality of the imposter syndrome that tightens its grip amid underperformance. In more extreme cases, my work involves supporting students whose severe physical and/or mental illness prevent them from continuing their studies, an outcome that often requires the difficult but necessary decision to take a medical leave of absence.

Among the more challenging aspects of my work is to help medical students who have engaged in unprofessional behaviours. Building on principles of resilience and self-compassion, I try to help students maintain accountability while orienting them towards growth and improvement and away from the shame that may occur when their identities become anchored in their indiscretions and mistakes.

My work involves helping students plan: to consider – and even dream about – what their lives will hold in the future. So often, our conversations about career choices and personal values intersect with themes of wellness. What kind of physician will I become? Will the rigours of training as "X" type of physician be worth it in the end? What, outside of work, will I have time to do in this profession? What will I be able to value and accomplish in my life? These questions both hinge on and deeply impact students' wellness. As they traverse the constant push and pull of pursuing medical careers while striving for health and happiness, I frequently remind them that their path may include turbulence, and that this can be a normal – albeit challenging – part of living well.

Critically, my work days include meeting students in some of their most joyous moments. This includes standing at the medical school entrance as they enter on their first day; placing their white coats as they take the initial oath of the profession of medicine; celebrating their successful residency match; and placing their doctoral hood at the end of their medical training. While outward excitement abounds in these moments, there pulsates the unspoken beauty of having quietly guided learners to the finish line of medical school despite tremendous obstacles, setbacks, and trials. In this beauty is wellness, that which was born, cultivated, and reinforced through both trial and triumph. In this beauty also exists apprehension for what comes next: the daunting years of residency training, where the trials and triumphs grow in magnitude. But in this moment on that graduation stage, there is no greater treasure than to see such joy and accomplishment embodied.

Supporting Learner Well-Being: A Clinical Psychologist/Family Medicine Behaviouralist Perspective

It is the second week of the month, and I am leading our monthly intern support group. It is midway through the academic year, and I pose a simple question for the residents in attendance: "How is everyone doing?"

Recollections and lamentations fill the air:

"I got treated like I was the nurse again this week. Second time this month."

"I received conflicting advice from two attendings. That was fun."

"I was so tired I fell asleep in the gym a few days ago."

"I started to cry in the precepting office and now everyone thinks I'm having a mental break down. I was just frustrated!"

"I am over being the new guy on the floor. Whenever I get my feet under me, the rotation is over and I start from scratch. It's exhausting."

Other residents empathize; some nod in solidarity. They share similar stories. I listen, validate, try to offer some cognitive restructuring when I can. But it's hard: all the psychological support, cognitive restructuring, and validation I can muster won't change a simple fact: the system in which these interns work and learn fundamentally antagonizes their attempts to be well.

– Andrada Neacsiu, Family Medicine Residency Behaviouralist

I (Andrada) am a builder of a resident wellness program. As a clinical psychologist and behaviouralist with approximately one-third of my time dedicated to a family medicine residency, my role is to promote resident wellness. I constantly scour all possible chances to apply my skills to that end, often with positive effect. However, many of the lamentations expressed in the support group above would be best addressed through sweeping, system-wide change, an idealistic goal that is well outside my individual sphere of influence. As a result, I work hard to validate the limitations of residents' ability to work within the current system, while simultaneously pushing them to adopt more effective ways of thinking, regulating emotions, and achieving self-care. The work of achieving this challenging goal most often occurs in 1:1 meetings, after-hours phone calls, and small support groups, its profundity, intensity, and intimacy invisible to anyone outside of the residents and me.

Prior to assuming this role, I expected to be something akin to a crisis worker: intervening with validation, problem solving, and skills in the height of distress. I also envisioned reducing such distress by teaching resilience skills and offering outlets for emotional expression. I do believe these aspects of my job are important and helpful. Nevertheless, I am consistently faced with barriers that I had not anticipated. First is the problem of measurement. How do we quantify wellness in medical education? I asked residents to periodically complete just about every self-report instrument I could find. What I learned – and all I learned – is that residents are generally not well and do worse in the winter. Not captured were the more subtle changes that I *observed* in how residents approached distress, thought about difficult situations, or accepted systemic shortcomings. Also not captured was clarity on what being "well" looks like in residency. In the current system, being well in residency involves, to some extent, fatigue, distress, disappointment, and lack of work-life balance. But what degree of stress is necessary for successful training and when do these stressors become too much? Even our best, most validated measures cannot capture this nuance. Therein lies some of the invisible work I do in support of resident wellness: attempting to determine what being well means to each individual I support.

Second, I have been surprised by how much of my work attends to the moral injury residents express at the hands of the systems in which they work and learn. Moral injury is defined as the distress experienced when one goes against their values or moral compass or witness others doing so.[32] Residents report recurrent distress when systemic limitations prevent them from providing the care patients deserve. Short visits, lack of protected time for asynchronous communication, systemic racism, politicization of healthcare, and other barriers impede integration of residents' own values and standards into the care of their patients. I intervene on moral injury by helping residents gain clarity on their professional values, understand how some values may come into conflict (e.g., helping as many people as one can versus providing in-depth, extensive care to every patient), and adopt skills for navigating such conflicts. I help them work towards acceptance of the fact that some situations require negotiating their values while trying to simultaneously empower them to advocate for change in the system that generates this tension.

Finally, it is difficult to build a program of wellness in a system that has historically trained and supported trainees from highly represented backgrounds who have little distraction from the outside world. The system's rigidity is particularly imposing for those whose learning abilities, sociocultural backgrounds, trauma histories, and/or financial limitations require adaptation and accommodation. It is within this imposing system that residents, at risk of perceiving that they are the problem that needs to change, are pressured to assimilate to the dominant norms from which they differ. This may be confusing to residents, who may wonder if their struggle comes from the normative difficulty of growth in medical training or from being a rose in a tulip garden and trying, or being forced, to become a tulip.

Concluding Thoughts

The work of these two individuals – whose contributions are anything but invisible – highlights the fundamental value of promoting learner *engagement* with the challenges inherent in learning medicine rather than simply seeking solutions. Facilitating such engagement requires patience, dedication, and curiosity, as well as a willingness to meet students where they are while guiding them to higher levels of achievement. This journey through medical education, while tumultuous at times, can be exhilarating, vitalizing, and awe-inspiring. Helping medical learners harness that wonder while supporting the hierarchy of needs that defines their humanity and fuels their well-being requires the work of a thousand ... and countless more.

Additional Reading

Bynum, W.E., Varpio, L., and Teunissen, P. 2021. Why impaired wellness may be inevitable in medicine, and why that may not be a bad thing. *Medical Education*, 55(1), 16–22. https://doi.org/10.1111/medu.14284

Bynum, W.E., Varpio, L., Lagoo, J., and Teunissen, P.W. 2021. "I'm unworthy of being in this space": the origins of shame in medical students. *Medical Education*, 55(2), 185–97. https://doi.org/10.1111/medu.14354

Bynum, W.E., Jackson, J.A., Varpio, L., and Teunissen, P. 2023. Shame at the gates of medicine: a hermeneutic exploration of pre-medical students' experiences of shame. *Academic Medicine*, 98(6), 709–16. https://doi.org/10.1097/ACM.0000000000005152

References

1. Bynum, W.E., Jackson, J.A., Varpio, L., and Teunissen, P. 2023. Shame at the gates of medicine: a hermeneutic exploration of pre-medical students' experiences of shame. *Academic Medicine*, 98(6), 709–16. https://doi.org/10.1097/ACM.0000000000005152

2. Lin, K.Y., Anspach, R.R., Crawford, B., Parnami, S., Fuhrel-Forbis, A., and De Vries, R.G. 2014. What must I do to succeed? Narratives from the US premedical experience. *Social Science & Medicine*, 119, 98–105. https://doi.org/10.1016/j.socscimed.2014.08.017

3. Bynum, W.E., Varpio, L., Lagoo, J., and Teunissen, P.W. 2021. "I'm unworthy of being in this space": the origins of shame in medical students. *Medical Education*, 55(2), 185–97. https://doi.org/10.1111/medu.14354

4. Bynum, W.E., Teunissen, P., and Varpio, L. 2021. In the "shadow of shame": a phenomenological exploration of the nature of shame experiences in medical students. *Academic Medicine*, 96(11S), S23–30. https://doi.org/10.1097/ACM.0000000000004261

5. Brennan, N., Corrigan, O., Allard, J., Archer, J., Barnes, R., Bleakley, A., Collett, T., and de Bere, S.R. 2010. The transition from medical student to junior doctor: today's experiences of tomorrow's doctors. *Medical Education*, 44(5), 449–58. https://doi.org/10.1111/j.1365-2923.2009.03604.x

6. O'Brien, B.C. 2018. What to do about the transition to residency? Exploring problems and solutions from three perspectives. *Academic Medicine*, 93(5), 681–4. https://doi.org/10.1097/ACM.0000000000002150

7. Bynum, W.E., Artino, A.R., Uijtdehaage, S., Webb, A.M.B., and Varpio, L. 2019. Sentinel emotional events: the nature, triggers, and effects of shame experiences in medical residents. *Academic Medicine*, 94(1), 85–93. https://doi.org/10.1097/ACM.0000000000002479

8. Gan, R., and Snell, L. 2014. When the learning environment is suboptimal: exploring medical students' perceptions of "mistreatment." *Academic Medicine*, 89(4), 608–17. https://doi.org/10.1097/ACM.0000000000000172

9. Leape, L.L., Shore, M.F., Dienstag, J.L., Mayer, R.J., Edgman-Levitan, S., Meyer, G.S., and Healy, G.B. 2012. Perspective: a culture of respect, part 1:

the nature and causes of disrespectful behavior by physicians. *Academic Medicine*, 87(7), 845–52. https://doi.org/10.1097/ACM.0b013e318258338d

10. Tsuei, S.H., Lee, D., Ho, C., Regehr, G., and Nimmon, L. 2019. Exploring the construct of psychological safety in medical education. *Academic Medicine*, 94(11S), S28–35. https://doi.org/10.1097/ACM.0000000000002897

11. Frank, E., Carrera, J.S., Stratton, T., Bickel, J., and Nora, L.M. 2006. Experiences of belittlement and harassment and their correlates among medical students in the United States: longitudinal survey. *BMJ*, 333(7570), 682. https://doi.org/10.1136/bmj.38924.722037.7C

12. Hu, Y.Y., Ellis, R.J., Hewitt, D.B., Yang, A.D., Cheung, E.O., Moskowitz, J.T., Potts, J.R. 3rd, et al. 2019. Discrimination, abuse, harassment, and burnout in surgical residency training. *New England Journal of Medicine*, 381(18), 1741–52. https://doi.org/10.1056/NEJMsa1903759

13. Rees, C.E., and Monrouxe, L.V. 2011. "A morning since eight of just pure grill": a multischool qualitative study of student abuse. *Academic Medicine*, 86(11), 1374–82. https://doi.org/10.1097/ACM.0b013e3182303c4c

14. Heru, A., Gagne, G., and Strong, D. 2009. Medical student mistreatment results in symptoms of posttraumatic stress. *Academic Psychiatry*, 33(4), 302–6. https://doi.org/10.1176/appi.ap.33.4.302

15. Schuchert, M.K. 1998. The relationship between verbal abuse of medical students and their confidence in their clinical abilities. *Academic Medicine*, 73(8), 907–9. https://doi.org/10.1097/00001888-199808000-00018

16. Puthran, R., Zhang, M.W., Tam, W.W., and Ho, R.C. 2016. Prevalence of depression amongst medical students: a meta-analysis. *Medical Education*, 50(4), 456–68. https://doi.org/10.1111/medu.12962

17. Dyrbye, L.N., West, C.P., Satele, D., Boone, S., Tan, L., Sloan, J., and Shanafelt, T.D. 2014. Burnout among U.S. medical students, residents, and early career physicians relative to the general U.S. population. *Academic Medicine*, 89(3), 443–51. https://doi.org/10.1097/ACM.0000000000000134

18. Holm, M., Tyssen, R., Stordal, K.I., and Haver, B. 2010. Self-development groups reduce medical school stress: a controlled intervention study. *BMC Medical Education*, 10, 23. https://doi.org/10.1186/1472-6920-10-23

19. Quek, T.T., Tam, W.W., Tran, B.X., Zhang, M., Zhang, Z., Ho, C.S., and Ho, R.C. 2019. The global prevalence of anxiety among medical students: a meta-analysis. *International Journal of Environmental Research and Public Health*, 16(15), 2735. https://doi.org/10.3390/ijerph16152735

20. Busireddy, K.R., Miller, J.A., Ellison, K., Ren, V., Qayyum, R., and Panda, M. 2017. Efficacy of interventions to reduce resident physician burnout: a systematic review. *Journal of Graduate Medicine Education*, 9(3), 294–301. https://doi.org/10.4300/JGME-D-16-00372.1

21. Daya, Z., and Hearn, J.H. 2018. Mindfulness interventions in medical education: a systematic review of their impact on medical student stress,

depression, fatigue and burnout. *Medical Teacher*, 40(2), 146–53. https://
doi.org/10.1080/0142159X.2017.1394999

22. Krasner, M.S., Epstein, R.M., Beckman, H., Beckman, H., Suchman, A.L.,
Chapman, B., Mooney, C.J., and Quill, T.E. 2009. Association of an educational program in mindful communication with burnout, empathy, and
attitudes among primary care physicians. *Journal of the American Medical
Association*, 302(12), 1284–93. https://doi.org/10.1001/jama.2009.1384

23. Simard, A.A., and Henry, M. 2009. Impact of a short yoga intervention
on medical students' health: a pilot study. *Medical Teacher*, 31(10), 950–2.
https://doi.org/10.3109/01421590902874063

24. Slavin, S.J., Schindler, D.L., and Chibnall, J.T. 2014. Medical student mental
health 3.0: improving student wellness through curricular changes. *Academic
Medicine*, 89(4), 573–7. https://doi.org/10.1097/ACM.0000000000000166

25. Walsh, A.L., Lehmann, S., Zabinski, J., Truskey, M., Purvis, T., Gould, N.F.,
Stagno, S., and Chisolm, M.S. 2019. Interventions to prevent and reduce
burnout among undergraduate and graduate medical education trainees:
a systematic review. *Academic Psychiatry*, 43(4), 386–95. https://doi.org
/10.1007/s40596-019-01023-z

26. Shiralkar, M.T., Harris, T.B., Eddins-Folensbee, F.F., and Coverdale, J.H. 2013.
A systematic review of stress-management programs for medical students.
Academic Psychiatry, 37(3), 158–64. https://doi.org/10.1176/appi.ap.12010003

27. Bynum, W.E., Varpio, L., and Teunissen, P. 2021. Why impaired wellness
may be inevitable in medicine, and why that may not be a bad thing.
Medical Education, 55(1), 16–22. https://doi.org/10.1111/medu.14284

28. Coentre, R., and Gois, C. 2018. Suicidal ideation in medical students:
recent insights. *Advances in Medical Education and Practice*, 9, 873–80.
https://doi.org/10.2147/AMEP.S162626

29. Aach, R.D., Girard, D.E., Humphrey, H., McCue, J.D., Reuben, D.B., Smith,
J.W., Wallenstein, L., and Ginsburg, J. 1992. Alcohol and other substance abuse
and impairment among physicians in residency training. *Annals of Internal
Medicine*, 116(3), 245–54. https://doi.org/10.7326/0003-4819-116-3-245

30. McBeth, B.D., Ankel, F.K., Ling, L.J., Asplin, B.R., Mason, E.J., Flottemesch,
T.J., and McNamara, R.M. 2008. Substance use in emergency medicine
training programs. *Academic Emergency Medicine*, 15(1), 45–53. https://doi
.org/10.1111/j.1553-2712.2007.00008.x

31. Arnedt, J.T., Owens, J., Crouch, M., Stahl, J., and Carskadon, M.A. 2005.
Neurobehavioral performance of residents after heavy night call vs
after alcohol ingestion. *Journal of the American Medical Association*, 294(9),
1025–33. https://doi.org/10.1001/jama.294.9.1025

32. Čartolovni, A., Stolt, M., Scott, P.A., and Suhonen, R. 2021. Moral injury in
healthcare professionals: a scoping review and discussion. *Nursing Ethics*,
28(5), 590–602. https://doi.org/10.1177/0969733020966776

Conclusion

22 In Conclusion: Let the Song Continue

LARA VARPIO, ANNE MAHALIK,
AND ANNA MACLEOD

If you have ever had the opportunity to sing as part of a choir, you know that successfully coordinating many voices into a harmonious whole is no simple task. It requires teamwork, active listening, concentration, and discipline. We draw the parallel between the silent work of many different people in medical education and choirs to highlight the fact that the field we call medical education comprises many different roles. Some roles receive a lot of attention in our field – clinician educators, researchers, institutional leaders, etc. These are roles that – to draw on our analogy – are given solos and so stand in front of and apart from the choir. In contrast, others are given little heed. These are the voices that do the hard work of maintaining the harmonies, intonations, and rhythm of the song so that the soloist can shine. These are the roles that we highlight in this book. Not the anatomist who leads the undergraduate anatomy class, but the anatomy technician who makes the class possible. Not the keynote speaker of the academic conference, but the conference conveners who make those conferences a welcoming home for the community. Not the medical school and academic teaching hospital leaders, but the administrators whose work supports and enables those leaders. Our intention with this book is to acknowledge and celebrate these roles – these silent voices – who are vital to the medical education enterprise. Without these individuals, medical schools and academic teaching hospitals would shutter; the entire enterprise would end. And yet, these people, these roles are generally ignored, overlooked, and silenced. We hope that by underscoring their contributions in this book, we contribute to a new appreciation for the influence they have – for the music they both make and make possible.

We organized this book into three sections to draw attention to the many ways that these unacknowledged roles are present in, and foundational to, medical education. In Section One, we focused on education delivery and the people who silently but actively engage in the training of future physicians – be it at the undergraduate level (e.g., anatomy technicians, simulated patients, test administrators, or community engagement facilitators) or at the graduate level (e.g., auxiliary nurses). We concentrated on those who contribute to the assembly of evidence in Section Two. Evidence that supports the running of the educational institutions (e.g., program evaluators and equity, diversity, and inclusion officers) and that contributes to the development of new knowledge (e.g., graduate students, librarians, conference conveners, and research funders) is crucial to the success of our field and made possible because of the work done in roles that are often unseen. Finally, Section Three addressed broader institutional concerns that influence medical education. The work conducted in support of individuals in the community (e.g., faculty development coordinators, workplace well-being staff, administration staff) and of the broader enterprise (e.g, technology support professionals, accreditation officers) ensures that structures and processes function as needed. Across all three sections and each chapter therein, it was important to us to include the voice of individuals who work in these silent roles. Therefore, in each chapter you heard the words of the people who have long been anonymous. In their stories you will hear their joy, frustrations, trials, and successes. We hope that readers find their words as moving as we have.

We hope it has become clear that medical education is, in fact, built on layers of work: some is visible, familiar, and well-valued, but some is very much less visible. These layers of work are, in fact, what make medical schools places of competence, caring, and character. What's interesting is when we *actually talked to people* about their work, we learned that their everyday challenges and the things that fill their days are so much more complex than what is reflected in a formal job description. This is the invisible work – but it was also in these moments that people seemed to find personal meaning in their roles. These were the tasks that seemed to be central to how people actually thought about their work, and about themselves as contributors to medical education. This was where they found joy and satisfaction, where they were able to shine. But it could also be the source of frustration and dissatisfaction. And because of that, we offer this volume as a space to listen to these stories. To hear these voices.

Imagine we had asked you a question before reading this book: what is the work of medical education? You likely would have answered quite straight forwardly: to educate physicians. Our hope is that although the answer to that question may not have changed, you now have a much better understanding of how that work is accomplished. Medical education is, in fact, a chorus. It includes a host of people, skills, and their multiple sets of expertise, certainly. But the choir also includes their emotions, their goals, their feelings about this complex enterprise of medical education, and their hopes. We believe this chorus of pedagogical partners sets the foundation for medical education and allows us to grow, improve, learn, and innovate when it comes to education. It allows us to sing more beautifully than we ever could have imagined.

We also acknowledge that the roles and voices that we highlight in this book are not all-inclusive. There are many others who warrant inclusion and attention but who are not included here. For instance, the work of building and custodial services staff are not presented. This absence is not a result of a lack of attention or interest. We sought out authors who felt comfortable addressing the vital work of people in these roles. We searched the literature to find scholars who had already addressed this contribution and who might be willing to give voice to these people in our book. Unfortunately, despite our best efforts, we were unable to find much that addressed building and custodial services in the peer-reviewed literature, nor were we able to secure authors to write about the people doing that work. And yet, we know – both anecdotally but also from the popular press – that janitorial work was critically important during the COVID-19 pandemic, for example. We regret that these voices – and so many others – are not part of this book.

Across all of the chapters in this volume, one theme resonates deeply: the need to acknowledge and investigate the contributions made to the field of medical education by the individuals doing the invisible work in each of the roles we highlight. It is clear from the stories narrated in this book that these people are vitally important to the education of future physicians. Licensed practice nurses (Chapter 8) teach learners strategies for surviving and excelling in different clinical contexts. Simulated patients (Chapter 4) and community engagement facilitators (Chapter 7) help learners appreciate how their clinical actions impact the lives of real patients. Graduate students (Chapter 11) and librarians (Chapter 12) are part of the teams of people needed to continue to advance the medical knowledge that learners will be required to harness for patient care. Even the learners themselves (Chapter 16) carry the weight of invisible work. And yet, despite their contributions, these individuals are largely ignored in our community's discussion of the work required to train future physicians. These individuals deserve our attention. Their contributions deserve recognition.

It's worth reiterating that so much of medical education occurs not in classrooms, but in real-life clinical settings. Workplace-based learning – where students are participating, as learners, in patient care; navigating team dynamics; and contributing to the routines of clinical life – is foundational to becoming a physician. But this learning depends on a chorus of people and their multiple roles: not just attending physicians and residents, but also administrators orienting learners to their schedules, preceptors adjusting their workflow to make space for questions, patients generously sharing their time, and countless others quietly ensuring the conditions for learning are in place. The workplace is a classroom – and invisible work is its scaffolding.

We conclude by reminding readers that people, and their work, matter. The people who keep medical schools running are many, and as this volume has made clear, they have so much expertise. However, it's easy not to see or hear them. In some cases, it's frankly easy to not notice them. But as this book has made clear, everyone wants to be seen and heard. We know from the literature in the sociology of work that being an invisible worker is exhausting.[1] It has been linked to burnout and stress,[2] particularly for those who are doing the work without recognition[3] or appropriate compensation.[3] Not seeing, not listening, not making the space to hear these stories has serious implications – for the individual workers, certainly, but also for the broader institution of medical education as it struggles with turnover and a sense of low morale.[3] The cycle continues, but we believe listening to the chorus is one important way to break that cycle.

Remember that medical education is a collective endeavour, ideally experienced as a harmonious choir. And we suggest that no matter what you're working on, take a moment and think about the diversity of people who are involved. Reflect upon who, in your institution, may have expertise to contribute, a perspective to share, an experience to consider. We implore you to challenge your assumptions about who ought to be involved. Whether you're working on curriculum, research, or an institutional project, think broadly about what expertise counts and could potentially make a meaningful contribution. And most importantly, make the space to talk with people. To hear about their work and their contributions to medical education.

For us, this book will be successful if it lands in the hands of leaders and community members in medical education, and if it spurs those individuals to recognize and appreciate the work of the many people who are part of the field and institutions of medical education. We would like to see our community recognize the specialized skills wielded by people in these roles. We hope to see their dedication more broadly respected and valued. Indeed, we hope that this book is a paean – i.e., a song of praise and thanksgiving – for those whose contributions to medical education have not been heard. We hope this book makes audible the chorus of silent voices of medical education's unsung heroes.

References

1. Star, S.L., and Strauss, A. 1999. Layers of silence, arenas of voice: the ecology of visible and invisible work. *Computer Supported Cooperative Work, 8*, 9–30. https://doi.org/10.1023/A:1008651105359
2. Crain, M., Poster, W., and Cherry, M., (eds.). 2016. *Invisible Labor: Hidden Work in the Contemporary World*. University of California Press.
3. Xiaoming, Y., Ma, B.J., Chang, C.L., and Shieh, C.J. 2014. Effects of workload on burnout and turnover intention of medical staff: A study. *Studies on Ethno-medicine*, 8(3), 229–37. https://doi.org/10.31901/24566772.2014/08.03.04

Contributors

Ralph Alberto-Marmol is a second-year medical student in the Vagelos College of Physician and Surgeons at Columbia University in New York City, USA. He is also the Community Relations and Social Work head at CoSMO, a student-run free medical clinic, and the co-chair for the orthopaedic surgery interest group at Columbia.

Louise Allen PhD, GradCertEdDes, BNutrDiet (Hons) is both a dietitian and an academic in health professions education. As a dietitian she has prior experience as a clinical dietitian and now works in a regulatory role for Dietitians Australia. As an academic she is a postdoctoral fellow in the Department of Medical Education at the University of Melbourne, Australia, and has experience with a range of research methods, focusing more recently on qualitative research; her areas of research include continuing professional development, evaluation, competency standards, advanced credentialing, and selection.

Jonathan Amiel MD is Director, Office of Professionalism and Inclusion in the Learning Environment, NewYork-Presbyterian, New York City, USA, and Adjunct Lecturer in Psychiatry and Behavioral Health at Stanford University School of Medicine, Stanford, California, USA.

Andrea M. Barker MPAS, PA-C is Director of the Center of Excellence in Musculoskeletal Care and Education and Co-director of the Advanced Fellowship in Health Professions Education Evaluation and Research at the Salt Lake City Veterans Affairs Healthcare Center, and Adjunct Assistant Professor of Physician Assistant Education and Sciences at the University of Utah, Salt Lake City, Utah, USA. As a clinician educator and program director, she has collaborated with many technology professionals including instructional designers, AV experts, and network specialists.

Erin Barry MS is an Assistant Professor of Anesthesiology, Military and Emergency Medicine, and Health Professions Education at the Uniformed Services University, Bethesda, Maryland, USA. With over a decade of experience in health professions education, she has served in a variety of technology-forward roles – including audio-visual specialist, instructional designer, and learning management system administrator – partnering with interprofessional teams to enhance medical training and curriculum delivery.

Beth Barron MD is Professor of Medicine and Course Director of Foundations of Medicine Tutorials at the Vagelos College of Physicians and Surgeons at Columbia University Medical Center, New York, USA.

Michael J. Battistone MD is Director of the Advanced Fellowship in Health Professions Education, Evaluation and Research, and Co-director of the Center of Excellence in Musculoskeletal Care and Education at the George E. Wahlen Veterans Affairs Medical Center in Salt Lake City, Utah, USA, and Professor of Medicine in the Division of Rheumatology at the University of Utah, Salt Lake City. With over 30 years of experience across the continuum of medical education, he has experienced the evolution of both curriculum delivery and technology professionals' roles within this changing landscape.

Kimberly Birdsall MPH is a public health professional with over 25 years of experience across multiple disciplines, including work in the private, government, religious, and non-profit sectors. Ms. Birdsall's commitment to advance health equity and address the social determinants of health comes from a passion for service and core belief of treating everyone with dignity and respect, as exemplified by her late parents. She is dedicated to working in partnerships to build communities and systems which give everyone an opportunity to live a healthy and happy life.

Kiranjit K. Brar MS is Director of Evaluation and Instructional Development, Office of Medical Education, Stanford School of Medicine, Stanford University, Stanford, California, USA.

Megan E.L. Brown MBBS, PhD is a Senior Research Associate at Newcastle University, UK.

Sarah Burm PhD an Associate Professor in Continuing Professional Development and Medical Education at Dalhousie University in Halifax, Nova Scotia, Canada.

Jamiu O. Busari MD, PhD is an Associate Professor of Medical Education at Maastricht University, the Netherlands; Adjunct Professor and Scientist, Institute for Disability and Rehabilitation Research at Ontario Tech University, Canada; and a consultant pediatrician at the Horacio Oduber Hospital, Aruba.

William E. Bynum MD, PhD is an Associate Professor of Family Medicine in Duke University's Department of Family Medicine and Community Health, Durham, North Carolina, USA. Will researches how medical learners experience the emotion of shame during their training. He is the co-founder and co-director of The Shame Lab, which advances healthy engagement with shame in professional practice.

Cristina Costache MBBS is a paediatrics trainee and a doctoral student at the University of Manchester, UK.

Michal Divney LCSW is the Senior Manager of Community Engaged Medical Education at the Hackensack Meridian School of Medicine, Nutley, New Jersey, USA. She is a licensed clinical social worker with more than 20 years' experience of non-profit counselling and management in organizational cultural competence, continuous quality improvement, trauma counselling, and program development. Michal seeks to provide medical students with personalized connections in the community as a way to shape their perspectives and ability to effectively work with people from diverse lived experiences.

Carolyn Doyle is the Director, Admissions, Faculty of Medicine, Dalhousie University in Halifax, Nova Scotia, Canada.

Rachel H. Ellaway PhD is Professor in Community Health Sciences and Director of the Office of Health and Medical Education Scholarship at the Cumming School of Medicine at the University of Calgary, Calgary, Alberta, Canada. She is also editor-in-chief of the journal *Advances in Health Sciences Education*.

Kevin W. Eva PhD is Associate Director and Scientist, Centre for Health Education Scholarship and Professor and Director of Education Research and Scholarship, Department of Medicine, University of British Columbia, Vancouver, British Columbia, Canada.

Gabrielle M. Finn PhD is Associate Vice President for Teaching, Learning, and Students, and Professor of Medical Education at the University of Manchester, UK.

Jason Frank MD, MA(Ed), FRCP, FAOA(hon) is Professor in the Department of Emergency Medicine and Director of the Centre for Innovation in Medical Education at University of Ottawa, Ottawa, Ontario, Canada.

Farah Friesen MI is Manager, Research and Knowledge Mobilization, Centre for Advancing Collaborative Healthcare and Education (CACHE), University of Toronto and University Health Network, Toronto, Ontario, Canada.

Neil Gesundheit MD, MPH is the Senior Associate Dean for Medical Education, George Deforest Barnett Founders Professor of Medicine and Professor (Teaching) of Medicine (Endocrinology), Stanford School of Medicine, Stanford University, Stanford, California, USA.

Gareth Gingell PhD is an Assistant Professor in the Department of Medical Education at Dell Medical School at the University of Texas, Austin, Texas, USA, and is an alumnus of the STEM Education Program there. His research focuses on race, equity, and power in health professions spaces.

Adam Hain DET, MAEd is the Associate Director of Instructional Development, Office of Medical Education, Stanford School of Medicine, Stanford University, Stanford, California, USA.

Marlies Hanssen-Bude is the retired coordinator of the secretariat of the Department of Pediatrics and its outpatient clinic at Zuyderland Hospital in Heerlen, the Netherlands. During this time, she also was the Program Administration Coordinator for the Paediatrics clerkship and residency training programs at the same hospital.

Mariam Hayward is Director, Inclusive Research Excellence and Impact, Western Research, Western University, London, Ontario, Canada.

Miriam Hoffman MD is Vice Dean for Academic Affairs at the new Hackensack Meridian School of Medicine, Nutley, New Jersey, USA. She has led the development, implementation, and continuous enhancement of the medical education program. Dr. Hoffman's goal is to align medical education curricula with health outcomes of populations and individuals, including addressing health inequities. Dr. Hoffman's focus on helping all populations achieve the highest health outcomes comes from her parents and grandparents, including her grandfather who was a general practitioner in the Bronx, laying the groundwork for Dr. Hoffman's career in family medicine.

Kimberley Hokin previously worked as Assessment Project Officer for the Department of Medical Education at the Melbourne Medical School, University of Melbourne, Australia.

Joseph A. Jackson MD is Associate Professor of Pediatrics in Duke University's Department of Pediatrics, Durham, North Carolina, USA. In addition to caring for pediatric patients in the outpatient setting, Joe serves as the Associate Dean for Student Affairs and directs the Duke School of Medicine Office of Student Affairs.

Terry Judd MD is Lead for Technology Enhanced Assessment in the Department of Medical Education at the Melbourne Medical School, University of Melbourne, Australia.

Renate Kahlke PhD is Assistant Professor, Department of Medicine, and a scientist at the McMaster Education Research, Innovation, and Theory Program, McMaster University, Hamilton, Ontario, Canada.

Reena Karani MD, MHPE is Professor (with tenure) of Medicine, Medical Education, and Geriatrics and Palliative Medicine, and Director of The Institute for Medical Education at the Icahn School of Medicine at Mount Sinai in New York City, New York, USA.

George Kovacs MD is an Emergency Physician and a Professor in the Department of Emergency Medicine and Medical Director for the Clinical Cadaver Program, Department of Medical Neuroscience, at Dalhousie University, Halifax, Nova Scotia, Canada.

Lorelei Lingard PhD is Professor, Department of Medicine and Faculty of Education, Western University, and Senior Scientist, Centre for Education Research and Innovation, Schulich School of Medicine and Dentistry, Western University, London, Ontario, Canada.

Victoria Luong MD is a research associate in Continuing Professional Development and Medical Education at Dalhousie University and a PhD Student in the Dalhousie Interdisciplinary PhD Program, Halifax, Nova Scotia, Canada.

Ricki Lynée is an award-winning actress, writer, producer, co-owner of Nuanse Entertainment, and a recipient of the 2021 All Stars Project/Castillo Theater Fellowship for Young Artists of Color. Ricki is also an actor-educator and works as a standardized patient participating in simulations, educating medical students and practising physicians in simulated patient programs in coordination with Columbia University Irving Medical College, Albert Einstein Medical College, Obstetric Emergency Simulations at Montefiore Medical Center, SUNY Downstate Medical College, and New York College of Podiatric Medicine, New York, USA.

Anna MacLeod PhD is Professor and Director of Education Research. She is the Assistant Dean for Student Affairs in the Faculty of Medicine, Dalhousie University, Halifax, Nova Scotia, Canada.

Anne Mahalik MAHSR is an evaluation specialist and research associate in the Office of Continuing Professional Development and Medical Education at Dalhousie University in Halifax, Nova Scotia, Canada.

Kate S. McOwen MSEd is the Senior Director of Medical Education Initiatives at the Association of American Medical Colleges in Washington, DC, USA.

Rhoda Meyer PhD is a lecturer in the Centre for Health Professions Education at the Faculty of Medicine and Health Sciences at Stellenbosch University, South Africa. As faculty development lead in the Department, she brings her lived experience of the role to the chapter, an experience that is framed by her background as a professional nurse, a nurse educator, and a qualified PhD health professions education scholar.

Andrada D. Neacsiu PhD is a clinical psychologist, Associate Professor in the Duke Department of Psychiatry and Behavioral Science, Director of Behavioral Health in the Duke Family Medicine Residency Program, and Director of the Brain Stimulation Research Center in Psychiatry, Duke University, Durham, North Carolina, USA. She is a National Institutes of Health–funded researcher focusing on the development of new interventions for difficulties with emotion regulation using neuroscience and technology.

Francisco Olmos-Vega MD, MHPE, PhD is Assistant Professor, Wenckebach Instituut voor Onderwijs en Opleiden, Universitair Medisch Centrum Groningen, the Netherlands, and Department of Anesthesiology, Pontificia Universidad Javeriana, Bogotá, Colombia

Pallavi Prathivadi PhD, MBBS, BMedSc (Hons), MMed, DCH, FRACGP is specialist academic general practitioner and Adjunct Senior Lecturer (Practice) at Monash University in Melbourne, Australia.

Andrea Rideout MD, FCFP is a family physician and the Assistant Dean for Admissions (Undergraduate Medical Education) at Dalhousie University in Halifax, Nova Scotia, Canada.

Carmela Rocchetti MD is a general internist and the Assistant Dean of Community Engaged Medical Education at the Hackensack Meridian School of Medicine, Nutley, New Jersey, USA. As a first-generation college and medical school graduate, her commitment to serving historically under-resourced populations stems from her family's personal hardships after immigrating from Italy. She has designed and developed the innovative human dimension course, inspiring students to address social determinants of health and become physician leaders who can make a lasting impact on communities.

Anna Ryan MBBS, PhD is Director of Assessment and Head of the Department of Medical Education at the Melbourne Medical School, University of Melbourne, Australia.

Anita Samuel PhD is an Associate Professor and Director of Distance Learning at the Center for Health Professions Education, Uniformed Services University, Bethesda, Maryland, USA. For over a decade, she has worked as a technology professional supporting faculty with their AV needs, providing learning management system support, and assisting with designing effective learning experiences. She has experienced stereotyping as "tech support" and recognizes the space she occupies as an invisible technology professional.

Robert Sandeski was a Licensed Funeral Director/Embalmer and the Manager of the Human Body Donation Program in the Faculty of Medicine at Dalhousie University, Halifax, Nova Scotia, Canada.

Stefanie S. Sebok-Syer PhD is an Assistant Professor (Research) of Emergency Medicine, Stanford School of Medicine, Stanford University, Stanford, California, USA.

Bassel Shanab is a medical student at the Yale School of Medicine, New Haven, Connecticut, USA, who is involved in basic needs research of health professional students as well as the social determinants of health in cardiovascular disease. He aspires to be a cardiologist with a focus on tailoring academic research to reduce systemic disparities in healthcare.

Jonathan Sherbino MD, MEd holds the William J Walsh Chair in Medical Education and is Professor, Department of Medicine, and Assistant

Dean of Health Professions Education Research, Faculty of Health Sciences, McMaster Health Education Research, Innovation & Theory (MERIT) Centre, McMaster University, Hamilton, Ontario, Canada.

Lindsey Sikora BSc (Hons), MISt, PhD(c) is the Head of Research Support (Health Sciences, Medicine, STEM). She is a medical librarian with over 10 years of experience in medicine, health sciences, information science and education, and is a doctoral candidate in medical education. She is also a methodologist in systematic and scoping reviews.

Liezl Smit MD, FCP, MMed, MSc, MPhil is a senior lecturer and paediatrician in the Department of Paediatrics and Child Health at the Faculty of Medicine and Health Sciences at Stellenbosch University, South Africa. She has a substantive teaching and leadership role within the medical program and offers a clinician's perspective on the importance of faculty development based on the influence that it has had on her own academic journey. She is currently registered for a PhD in health professions education.

Renée E. Stalmeijer PhD is an Associate Professor of Medical Education at the School of Health Professions Education and Department of Educational Development and Research at the Faculty of Health, Medicine, and Life Sciences at Maastricht University in the Netherlands.

Lisa Thurgur MD, FRCPC is Assistant Professor, Department of Emergency Medicine, University of Ottawa, Ottawa, Ontario, Canada.

Jacqueline Torti PhD is Assistant Professor, Department of Medicine and Faculty of Education, Western University, and Scientist, Centre for Education Research & Innovation, Schulich School of Medicine & Dentistry, Western University, London, Ontario, Canada

Sandy Tse MD, MEd, FRCPC is Assistant Professor, Departments of Pediatrics and Emergency Medicine, and Assistant Dean CQI and Accreditation, Postgraduate Medical Education, University of Ottawa, Ottawa, Ontario, Canada.

Susan van Schalkwyk PhD is Professor Emeritus and former Executive Head of the Department of Health Professions Education at the Faculty of Medicine and Health Sciences at Stellenbosch University, South Africa.

Lara Varpio PhD is Professor in the Department of Pediatrics at the Perelman School of Medicine at the University of Pennsylvania and Co-Director of Research in Medical Education at The Children's Hospital of Philadelphia. Both institutions are located in Philadelphia, Pennsylvania, USA.

Jaymie Walker, MSc, MD is General Surgery Chief Resident in the Department of Surgery at the University of Calgary, Calgary, Alberta, Canada.

CDR Jason Weiner MC, USN is the Chair of the Department of Medicine at Naval Medical Center San Diego, California, USA, Clinical Associate Professor of Medicine at the Uniformed Services University, Bethesda, Maryland, USA, and Volunteer Clinical Assistant Professor at the University California San Diego Division of Rheumatology, Autoimmunity, and Inflammation. As a clinician educator, CDR Weiner has served as an Associate Program Director for the Internal Medicine Residency Program at Naval Medical Center San Diego and collaborates extensively across the healthcare educational spectrum in curriculum design, assessment and prototype development, and continuing professional development.

Tasha R. Wyatt PhD is Full Professor of Medicine and Health Professions Education, Department of Health Professions Education, Center for Health Professions Education at Uniformed Services University of the Health Sciences, Bethesda, Maryland, USA. She is a critical educational researcher who studies how systems of oppression affect the experiences of physicians and trainees in educational and clinical settings.

Jazmin Zuleta-García LPN is a licensed practice nurse at Hospital Universitario San Ignacio, Bogotá, Colombia.